CASE STUDIES OF MENTAL HEALTH PARAPROFESSIONALS

PARAPROFESSIONALS

Twelve Effective Programs

CASE STUDIES OF MENTAL HEALTH PARAPROFESSIONALS

Twelve Effective Programs

Sam R. Alley, Ph.D.

Judith Blanton, Ph.D.

Ronald E. Feldman, Ph.D.

Glenn David Hunter, Ph.D.

Michael Rolfson, M.A.

Social Action Research Center
San Rafael, California

HUMAN SCIENCES PRESS
72 Fifth Avenue   3 Henrietta Street
NEW YORK, NY 10011 ● LONDON, WC2E 8LU

Library of Congress Catalog Number 79-11081

ISBN: 0-87705-416-9

Printed in the United States of America
9 987654321

This project was funded by Grant #5-T41-MH 14487, provided by the Paraprofessional Manpower Development Branch, Division of Manpower and Training, National Institute of Mental Health.

Library of Congress Cataloging in Publication Data

Social Action Research Center.
  Case studies of mental health paraprofessionals.

  Bibliography: p.
  Includes index.
  1. Allied mental health personnel. 2. Mental health services. I. Alley, Sam. II. Title.
[DNLM: 1. Allied health personnel. 2. Community mental health services—Manpower—United States. WM21 P224]
RC440.2.S63 1979   610.69'53   79-11081
ISBN 0-87705-416-9

CONTENTS

FOREWORD

Although paraprofessional personnel have been involved in providing mental health services for as long as there have been organized systems of care, it was not until the early 1960s that their real and potential contributions became formally recognized. During that time, the National Institute of Mental Health, through its Experimental and Special Training Branch, funded a variety of paraprofessional training and utilization projects. In 1965, that Branch initiated a highly successful pilot Mental Health Associate of Arts degree support program. As a result of those initial efforts, there are now over 200 such programs in operation around the country. The Institute also made significant contributions to developing paraprofessional personnel through the Hospital Staff Development Program and through some early demonstration efforts by the Community Mental Health Services Support Branch.

By 1971, the Institute's recognition and acceptance of the importance of paraprofessionals in the delivery of mental health services had grown to the point that the New Careers Training Program was established as a separate and distinct entity within the Division of Manpower and Training Programs. The purpose of the program was to foster the development of paraprofessionals as service providers in the mental health field. In 1973, the New Careers Training Program was elevated to the status of a branch, to exist side by side with its sister branches in psychiatry, psychology, social work, nursing, continuing education, and experimental and special training.

In 1975, the New Careers Training Branch changed its name to the Paraprofessional Manpower Development Branch and issued new program guidelines which were more consistent with the Branch's expanded mandate. There were several reasons for the name change: (1) The term "Manpower Development" embodies more activities than just training; (2) the term "New Careers" had come to be associated with "pre-service" and "entry level" training; and (3) the change of the name reflected official sanction for the Branch to involve itself with the myriad of issues affecting paraprofessionals at various skill levels and in different settings. These changes set the stage for the Branch to deal with many of the major issues that needed attention. These issues included acceptance and effective utilization of paraprofessionals, worker certification, education and training program standards, competency identification and assessment, deinstitutionalization, continuing education, and needs assessment.

As a result of these changes and the expanded role of the Branch, two leadership questions emerged:

1. How could the Branch promote local and national recognition of the significant contributions of paraprofessionals as effective and efficient service providers, as well as foster the continued training of paraprofessionals and the overall development of the paraprofessional field?
2. How could the Branch demonstrate that the effective use of paraprofessionals can and should be an important strategy for meeting the additional service requirements for community mental health centers under Public Law 94-63?

In an attempt to address these questions, the Social Action Research Center was awarded a grant to develop and disseminate a variety of materials to increase the awareness of mental health practitioners, administrators, and policymakers about the real and potential effectiveness of paraprofessionals and to improve the efficient use of this significant resource. As a part of this grant, Social Action Research Center's Paraprofessional Utilization Project produced three significant volumes on paraprofessionals: *Paraprofessionals in Mental Health: An Annotated Bibliography, 1966 to 1977; Paraprofessionals in Mental Health: Theory and Practice;* and this collection of case studies of programs using paraprofessional staff to provide effective mental health services in community settings.

These case studies document the wide range of jobs in which paraprofessionals currently are working and the high quality of the services they are capable of providing. The programs in this volume are not unique, however. There are many other projects which also could serve as models for effective paraprofessional utilization. Yet, while there are few mental health programs which do not use paraprofessionals, there are still too many which fail to use their paraprofessional staff as effectively or efficiently as they might. We hope these case studies will help programs improve their use of staff members to meet their present and expanding client needs.

In our own experience in the field, we have also noted the problems mentioned in these case studies (lack of paraprofessional job mobility, low salaries, conflicts around status, need for improved pre-service and in-service training, etc.). Our Branch is attempting to deal with these issues through support for other projects involving competency-based education, development of career ladders, innovative training programs, and so forth. We hope that future mental health service programs will be able to benefit from these endeavors.

Paraprofessionals are an important, although often invisible, part of our mental health service system. Without them, many clients would not be served or would be served poorly. We hope that these descriptions of the tasks paraprofessionals are providing will help give this significant group the attention that it so well deserves.

Paraprofessional Manpower Development Branch

Donald L. Fisher
Vernon R. James
George W. White

ACKNOWLEDGMENTS

Many people and organizations contributed valuable assistance to the development of these case studies. The Paraprofessional Manpower Branch of the National Institute of Mental Health (NIMH), and in particular Vernon James, provided not only the funding for this undertaking but also important direction and encouragement. Don Fisher and George White of the Branch contributed helpful suggestions regarding format and content. Mary Bilstad, Vieva Monteau, and Carolyn Snowden were of great assistance in expediting the process of program operations. Referrals to many potential study sites were given by the NIMH regional offices and by many individuals working in the field of mental health. Andre Abecassis, Herbert Highstone, Karen Mann, Marge Mysyk, and Duane Welsch provided excellent support by editing, typing, and proofreading and by including many valuable suggestions for improving the readability of the studies.

Most of all we would like to acknowledge our great debt to the mental health programs whose work is being reported in this volume. Without exception, the program staff members made us feel welcome and answered our interminable questions cheerfully and openly. It is our hope that these case studies convey the enthusiasm that we found during our visits and that they effectively document the high quality of services being provided.

Chapter 1

INTRODUCTION

Paraprofessionals are an essential personnel resource in the provision of mental health services. Many drug, alcohol, and suicide prevention programs are administered and staffed primarily by paraprofessionals. Within hospital settings, paraprofessionals work as psychiatric technicians and nurses' assistants, demonstrating a high level of responsibility, especially when a milieu therapy approach is used. Community mental health centers, particularly those that emphasize an outreach approach, often depend heavily on paraprofessional staff members. Centers make use of paraprofessionals to provide such services as intake screening, crisis intervention, casefinding, case management, psychosocial rehabilitation, and outpatient counseling. It has been estimated (Brown, 1975) that up to 150,000 auxiliary mental health workers are presently employed in our hospitals, community mental health centers, clinics, day care facilities, residential treatment centers, and other multiservice facilities, both public and private. Steinberg, Freeman, Steele, Balodis, and Batista (1976) estimate that at least 30% of direct mental health services are furnished by paraprofessionals.

Paraprofessionals are sometimes viewed merely as a means of supplementing the activities of professionals and thereby offering services to a larger number of clients. However, paraprofessionals are also used to provide new mental health services in response to changing times and philosophies. Unencumbered by traditional role restraints, these workers have generated many innovations in response to the specific needs of their clients, and such contributions should be seen as complementary to professional activities.

The growth and development of community mental health centers were set in motion by federal legislation that, in 1963, provided construction funds (PL 88-164) and, in 1965, established staffing grants (PL 89-105). Numerous sources (e.g., Bloom, 1977) describe the resulting nationwide activities of the next dozen years. The amendments to this legislation, which culminated in the 1975 federal legislation (PL 94-63, Title III, including the Community Mental Health Center Amendments of 1975), were aimed in part at broadening the centers' efforts to combat social ills that result in individual emotional disorders (Bloom, 1977).

The 1975 legislation specifically expands the number of services required of a federally supported community mental health center (CMHC) from five to twelve. The original five services were inpatient, outpatient, emergency, day care, and consultation and education. In addition to these, a community mental health center must now provide follow-up, transitional and screening services, alcohol and drug abuse services, and services specifically tailored to children and the aging. This action by Congress led to the expansion of many programs within existing centers as well as to the development of a large number of new centers.

Preliminary investigation by the Paraprofessional Manpower Development Branch of NIMH indicated that many mental health center policymakers and staff were unaware of either alternative models of providing services to clients, or of the wide array of tasks in which paraprofessional staff have been successfully employed. This volume of case studies was developed as one aspect of a grant awarded by this Branch[1] and is designed to provide these policymakers and staff with examples of effective mental health programs employing paraprofessionals. We selected 12 programs, one in each service area, and describe the model of service delivery, how the individual program meshed with the rest of the center, and the historical development of both center and program. Since our particular focus is on the ways in which paraprofessionals can be used to improve services to clients, each chapter describes the tasks performed by paraprofessionals, and discusses how each program has resolved the critical issues of selection, recruitment, education, training, supervision, mobility, status, and morale. A concluding chapter examines the programs, seeking similarities that might be factors in their successful operation.

We hope that readers of this book will find ideas useful in planning new mental health programs or expanding current ones. We view these chapters not as detailed blueprints, but rather as architects' models. The programs described in this volume should introduce readers to the tremendous possibili-

---

[1]Two other volumes include a bibliography: *Paraprofessionals in mental health: An annotated bibliography from 1966 to 1977* and *Paraprofessionals in mental health: Theory and practice.*

ties inherent in the paraprofessional work force, and provide stimulation for the more effective employment of paraprofessional staff to meet the needs of our mental health clients.

SELECTION OF THE SITES VISITED

Essentially the same series of procedures was used to locate and select the programs in each of the 12 different service delivery areas. Three stages were involved: (1) gathering leads on centers or programs to be contacted; (2) calling individual centers or programs for detailed information; and (3) selecting candidate programs on the basis of a set of criteria.

The leads were obtained from personal visits, phone calls and letters to knowledgeable people in the mental health field, including various sources in Washington, D.C. Requests were made by mail to each of the 10 Department of Health, Education, and Welfare regional offices asking for possible sites in each service area. Those offices that did not respond were contacted by follow-up phone calls. Furthermore, we contacted relevant organizations such as the National Council of Community Mental Health Centers, people from universities who were considered to be expert in a specific service delivery area, and researchers who had visited a number of mental health centers.

Depending on the information received, we either contacted the director of the mental health center or called the program chief directly. During these telephone interviews we asked a long series of questions concerning general features of program service delivery and use of paraprofessionals. We also requested copies of any relevant written materials describing aspects of the program, such as grant applications, newspaper articles, and books authored by staff members.

In order to select the sites to be visited, we compared centers within each of the 12 categories against an array of criteria. The criteria on which choices were based follow.

Quality of Services

We selected programs that employed paraprofessional staff members in the provision of quality services to clients. General guidelines applicable to all programs were developed with the assistance of Judy Turner of the National Institute of Mental Health, Support Service Branch. Quality criteria specific to each service area were derived from guidelines developed by NIMH. What follows is a list of features that we looked for in all programs.

1. Maximum availability and accessibility of services.
2. Rapid formulation and implementation of treatment plans.
3. Systematic evaluation of treatment.

4. Good relationships between program and community, particularly with associated human service agencies.
5. Procedures to guarantee patient rights.
6. Orientation to a case management approach, with a primary clinician who maintains treatment responsibility through varying services.
7. Innovative treatment methodologies that remain consonant with sound mental health practices.
8. Use of an outreach approach when appropriate.
9. Emphasis on self-determination as a goal for clients.
10. Multiracial, bilingual staff when appropriate to treating diverse clientele.
11. Creation, whenever possible, of normalized rather than clinic-like treatment settings.

Use of Paraprofessionals

Good use of paraprofessionals was an important criterion in program selection. The subcriteria that follow were developed from an earlier analysis of mental health programs using paraprofessionals (Alley, Blanton, Churgin, & Grant, 1975).

1. Paraprofessionals are defined as regular paid employees with bachelor of arts degrees or less.
2. Paraprofessionals comprise a sizeable percentage of the service team (at least two full-time paraprofessionals).
3. Paraprofessionals work with staff members who represent a variety of disciplines.
4. A significant proportion of the program's service delivery is carried out by paraprofessionals.
5. Paraprofessional staff members have meaningful responsibilities.
6. Reasons for using paraprofessionals extend beyond cost; that is, there is an awareness of the unique experience and skills they bring to a program. In a good program, paraprofessional tasks go beyond supplementing professionals, and in addition broaden the types of services available.
7. Recruitment of staff members is oriented to the community served.
8. Selection procedures emphasize skills and experience rather than academic qualifications.
9. Ongoing training is emphasized, preferably with academic credit arranged at local colleges and universities.
10. Supervision, preferably of a formal nature, is regularly carried out.
11. A career ladder or other means for providing meaningful career mobility exists.
12. Ongoing evaluation exists in some form.
13. Mutual learning and interaction between professional and paraprofessional staff exists.

14.   Paraprofessionals are assisted and encouraged to continue their formal education, when appropriate.

Widely Applicable Models

We wanted to locate programs that would be useful as models for other programs and program planners, programs that would exemplify effective and innovative service delivery.

1.   We sought programs whose success did not depend primarily on the unusual skills or charismatic personalities of key individuals, but rather appeared to depend on more concrete organizational features. For example, programs which required the particular resources available only from a close connection with a major university were not selected, nor were programs whose functioning seemed dependent on the personality of the director.
2.   We sought a variety of philosophical approaches in the 12 sites selected. We were particularly interested in how innovative theories were put into practice.
3.   Programs were selected that had been established for some time. In certain relatively recently mandated service areas this was not possible, but we were wary of using programs in their first blush of success.
4.   We chose programs from different regions of the country, with diverse client populations in terms of urban versus suburban versus rural, poor versus middle class, and racial and ethnic variety.
5.   The program administration and staff had to be open to our time-consuming, service-interfering site visit. We explained in our telephone interviews that we would need to talk to every staff member for at least an hour, and perhaps spend considerably more time with some.

No program, of course, matched these ideal criteria exactly. However, we were pleased and excited to find that in every case the actual site visit confirmed the high opinion we had formed as the result of preliminary investigation. We hope that the following chapters convey our enthusiasm for the work being done by these programs.

REFERENCES

Alley, S. R., Blanton, J., Churgin, S., & Grant, J. D. New careers: Strategies for change in community mental health. JSAS *Catalog of Selected Documents in Psychology*, 1975, *5*, 260–261.

Bloom, B. *Community mental health: A general introduction.* Belmont, Calif.: Brooks-Cole, 1977.

Brown, B. S. *The training of mental health auxiliaries for mental health care.* Paper presented at the Annual Meeting of the Indian Psychiatric Society in Trivandrum, India, January, 1975.

Steinberg, S. S., Freeman, K. A., Steele, C. A., Balodis, I., & Batista, A. L. (University Research Corporation). *Information on manpower utilization, functions, and credentialing in community mental health centers* (contract no. ADM 45-74-158). Washington, D.C.: Department of Health, Education, and Welfare, National Institute of Mental Health, Division of Manpower and Training, 1976.

Chapter 2

AGING SERVICES

INTRODUCTION

Description of the Service Area

The 1975 Community Mental Health Center Amendments require that special attention be paid to the mental health needs of the elderly. While the elderly have always received care at community mental health centers, services appropriate to their special needs have been limited, and community mental health centers are now required to devote specific attention and resources to this population. To this end, community mental health centers should assign to a full-time staff person the responsibility for the development, implementation, and coordination of programs for the elderly. In addition, administrative and clinical staff members, as well as the necessary financial resources, should be made available for this purpose.

Programs for the elderly must include all the regular services of the center, but should gear them to the physical and emotional needs of this special client group. In addition to relevant cognitive, emotional, and social evaluation, diagnostic services must include a physical health assessment. Because elderly people often have difficulties reaching available services, it is important that the treatment services be accessible. Outreach services and home visits should be an integral part of programs for the elderly. Mental health services should be coordinated with agencies that provide assistance to elderly clients, in order to enhance continuity of care.

Selection of the Site Visited

Services oriented specifically to elderly clients were newly mandated by the 1975 Community Mental Health Center Amendments. We learned that many centers do not have special programs in this area, perhaps in part because these services have only recently been required.

The Aging Program of the Hillsborough Community Mental Health Center was recommended by Gene Cohen, M.D., of the department of Studies of Mental Health of the Aging, National Institute of Mental Health. After lengthy telephone conversations with program administrators and staff members, we decided to use the Hillsborough Center as the site for our chapter on aging services. This aging program provides, in accord with the 1975 guidelines, a wide variety of therapeutic, rehabilitative, and primarily outreach-oriented direct services to individual elderly clients. This program also provides consultation and education services to relevant community agencies.

The paraprofessional workers in the Hillsborough Aging Program have broad responsibilities in the provision of both direct and indirect services. The program has developed an excellent model of professional/paraprofessional teamwork that emphasizes the complementary nature of this relationship.

HILLSBOROUGH COMMUNITY MENTAL HEALTH CENTER: A CASE STUDY IN AGING SERVICES*

The Hillsborough Community Mental Health Center serves the residents of the catchment area in Tampa, Florida. The aging program, which will be described in this chapter, serves Hillsborough County residents over 55 years of age. This group comprises about 19% of the county's population.

The aging program component of the Hillsborough Community Mental Health Center is physically located within the main building of the center. The program provides direct services, consultation, education, and coordination services. It has a predominantly outreach orientation. The service delivery team is made up of five mental health technicians, all paraprofessionals, who are supported by a recreational therapist, an occupational therapist, and a social worker, all of whom work full time; a psychiatrist and an evaluator both

*Contact: Hillsborough Community Mental Health Center
        5707 North 22nd Street
        Tampa, Florida   33610
        813/237-3914
        Attention: Beverly Boe, Program Director

work half time, and a psychologist works 20% of the time. The program
director is a registered nurse who has past administrative experience.

The program carries over 200 open cases. During the last year 284 cases
were closed. The monthly average during the second half of the fiscal year
1975–76 was 515 direct service contacts, 280 coordination contacts, and 38
consultation contacts. The program's target group includes individuals aged
55 years and older who reside in the county and have need for mental health
services. In addition to direct services, a primary emphasis of the aging program is to provide consultation and coordination to the community health
organizations that provide the elderly with housing, food, medical care, and
social service.

Background

The Hillsborough Community Mental Health Center originated in 1947 as a
Planned Parenthood agency. Over the years the center has evolved from its
original purpose and has expanded to provide a variety of community services.
In 1966, services for adults and children were housed together in one building.
In 1972, a federal staffing grant allowed the center to expand to its present size.

The Hillsborough center has recently been reorganized. In the past, each
discipline—psychiatry, psychology, nursing, social work, and mental health
technicians—had its own hierarchy. The reorganization provides for grouping
by function with separate coordinators responsible for the three types of service: adult, child, and outreach. The outreach coordinator is responsible for
the program in aging, as well as for adult day treatment, a halfway house, the
alcohol abuse services, and three satellite centers.

Overall there are 135 nonadministrative staff members employed by the
center; 104 are professionals and 31 are paraprofessionals. The total budget for
the last fiscal year (1975–76) was just over $2,800,000. Professional salaries
amounted to $964,847, while the paraprofessionals received $146,205. The
average paraprofessional salary was $6,500.

The center's philosophy is to provide services related to mental health so
that clients will have alternatives to hospitalization in state-operated facilities.

The aging program was started on April 1, 1975, when a funding grant
was obtained from the Florida State Division of Mental Hygiene by a social
worker in the center, who then became the program's first director.

The reasons for beginning a new program as part of any community
mental health center are generally varied. The personal motivations of the
staff, the political climate, and the availability of funds all play a part in such
a decision. In this case, the community need for an aging program had been
recognized for some time by the Hillsborough Community Mental Health
Center. An aging program had been viewed as part of a future expansion, but
the unexpected availability of special funds allowed the center to hire additional staff for that purpose sooner than had originally been planned.

At first, the aging program was located in a nearby community church. The center director then moved it into the main facility of the center. The move, which occurred during the program's first year, was motivated by the financial difficulties that the center was facing. The use of available office space within the center reduced the operating costs of the program. In addition, the center's director was concerned that the aging program's separate physical location would contribute to a split between the program's staff members and the rest of the center.

During this same period, the center director replaced the original program director with the present program director. The move to the center's main building and the appointment of a new program director were attempts by the center director to better integrate the program into the rest of the center's operations.

Program Organization and Services

The paraprofessionals in the aging program at the Hillsborough Community Mental Health Center play a major role in providing direct services to clients. The professional staff members do provide some direct service, but they function more as support, supervision, and backup for the paraprofessionals. In addition to providing direct client service, each paraprofessional is assigned a specific area in which to develop expertise. For example, one paraprofessional is familiar with nursing homes, another understands boarding homes, a third works with the state hospital, a fourth consults, and so on. The paraprofessionals have become so knowledgeable that the professionals are turning to them for information about these areas.

Clients are encouraged to make use of the facilities of the aging program at the mental health center when they are appropriate. They can be screened by a paraprofessional and seen by the psychologist for an evaluation. In some cases the psychiatrist, along with a paraprofessional, sees an individual for therapy. The psychiatrist may also prescribe medication. Every client is given information about the medication prescribed. Periodically, the clients are asked what medication they are taking and what the dosage is; they are reminded if they have forgotten. The psychiatrist relies on the paraprofessionals to follow up in this area. They are able to help the clients get prescriptions filled and to monitor the clients while they take medications at home. The paraprofessionals have received training so that they are aware of adverse reactions or the need for increased dosage. The psychiatrist at Hillsborough has confidence in the paraprofessionals' abilities to assist him in this area. When indicated, the paraprofessionals also coordinate their treatment activities with those doctors outside the aging program who have medical responsibilities for the center's clients.

There are different types of groups available for the elderly clients at the center. The insight groups deal with the discovery of self. Clients who are not diagnosed as psychotic and who are verbal are encouraged to take part in these groups. There are also support groups oriented toward the solution of problems in the here and now. The paraprofessionals act as cotherapists in the insight groups and sometimes as sole therapists in the support groups. They usually begin doing cotherapy with a professional staff member and then graduate to the primary responsibility of leading a group when they have enough experience.

In addition to therapy groups, the program also offers activity groups which are run by the recreational and occupational therapists with the help of the paraprofessionals. Staff members feel it is important to design activities that do not condescend to, but are still within the capabilities of, these clients. They have developed a book of activities based on their cumulative experience. Physical exercise is incorporated into all activity groups; each group begins with some exercises, and clients are encouraged to exercise at home. Group field trips to scenic spots also are organized.

One paraprofessional staff member from the aging program works specifically with the state hospital, which is located 80 miles from Tampa. Of the 3,000 hospital patients, 220 come from the Tampa area. One goal of the aging program is to get these patients discharged from the state hospital and successfully reestablished in the community. To accomplish this goal, the paraprofessional has set up predischarge groups at the hospital. These groups are oriented toward the problems of reentry into the community and assist the client in speeding up the readiness for reenty. The hospital is adept at giving medication to the patients but has limited facilities for social interaction and therapy. Hospital personnel welcome the assistance of the aging program workers, although it has sometimes been difficult to get the hospital to follow through on necessary details.

Many of the patients at the state hospital do not want to leave. However, the predischarge groups are aimed at helping them overcome their fears. The paraprofessional also works with the families of these patients to prepare them for the client's discharge from the hospital and for their future responsibilities. The paraprofessional continues to work with the family of the client after discharge from the hospital.

Working with families is an important aspect of the paraprofessionals' task, for they provide the support and information necessary for the difficult undertaking of caring for an elderly relative. For example, one paraprofessional worked with a woman under the age of 55 whose elderly husband was sent to a nursing home and explained to her the nature of chronic brain syndrome and the medication procedures. The paraprofessional also helped the woman confront the feelings of grief and guilt that resulted when it was necessary to confine her husband. Often an explanation of the aging process serves to allay many fears of the family and equips them to better understand the situation.

The aging program continually emphasizes the concept of self-help by the client. It may be easier to do things for the clients, but it is felt that they are best served by being helped to do things for themselves whenever possible. It is important for elderly persons to learn to buy food, take care of their living space, get medical attention, and become more involved in daily activities in order to move in the direction of a healthy, more self-sufficient status.

The philosophy at the aging program is to decrease the emphasis on the direct services offered where possible, and to increase community consultation and coordination of existing services so that greater client coverage will be possible. Thus, the aim is to educate the nursing home staff, the retirement community staff, the hospital personnel, and the people of the community on how to better care for their elderly citizens. If community organizations are better coordinated, and if consultation leads to improved services, then greater, more effective client coverage can be accomplished.

Although this concept of working with community elements to improve care for the elderly is an excellent philosophy, it is difficult to put into practice. There is a strong desire by clients to continue receiving direct services. The elderly clients like the attention they receive from the paraprofessionals. The relationships that are established provide important sources of personal satisfaction and interest for them.

The nursing home, retirement community, and hospital staffs welcome the paraprofessionals and their novel programs and ideas. Their services tend to be looked on as a "free gift." The paraprofessionals try to define clearly their function as trainers and consultants. They initiate programs and model methods which can be taken over by the staff members of these agencies. The agency staff would then be responsible for continuing these programs and, hopefully, for beginning others. All too often, however, as soon as the aging program paraprofessional stops going to these agencies, the programs are not carried through and are allowed to perish.

In one nursing home, the aging program's director began a therapy group that she and a paraprofessional led together. The director then had the nursing home's activities director replace her, while the paraprofessional continued to assist. Success was finally achieved when the activities director began to lead the group on her own. Unfortunately, shortly afterward the activities director quit her job at the nursing home, and the process had to be undertaken anew. This example illustrates just one of the many difficulties inherent in this approach.

Issues in Service Delivery.   The question, "Who is a suitable client?" is typical for mental health programs. In the aging program, "suitable" implies that a client is able to be helped. Those clients who are severely physically disabled, impaired by organic pathology, psychotic, or who in other ways present little hope for rehabilitation are considered not suitable. One source of difficulty is that personnel from other Hillsborough center programs often refer *any* client over 55 to the aging staff as if age were the sole criterion. What must be guarded against is that so-called unsuitable clients may be allowed to "fall between the cracks" and may not receive appropriate help from anyone.

Outreach services, by definition, require that staff members spend the majority of their time in the community, away from the main facility and their immediate supervisors. The paraprofessionals do the bulk of outreach work in the aging program. They enjoy the full confidence of their program director and the professional staff. It should be noted that the possibility does exist for animosity to develop between outreach personnel and center staff. Those working in the main building throughout the day might be jealous of the apparent freedom of the outreach workers. The aging program occasionally makes use of the center's in-service training meetings to educate staff members from other programs as to the nature of the task of outreach workers. One purpose of this education is to diminish staff problems due to misunderstandings.

Transportation is a major difficulty in providing services to the elderly. Public transit in the Tampa area is considered poor, although there are some resources which furnish transportation available for the elderly, such as neighborhood service centers. In addition, clients on Social Security Insurance are eligible to receive transportation to and from the center. Arranging and coordinating transportation for a group of elderly clients is often extremely time consuming. Preparation for an activity may have to begin days in advance. The program uses vans to facilitate transportation, but getting elderly people in and out of them is sometimes an insurmountable challenge. One criterion for employment as a van driver in the aging program is that the employee be big and strong.

Staff members note the need for paraprofessional outreach workers to be aware of the total needs of their elderly clients. Elderly persons still have sexual feelings. This is often difficult for a person 20 to 30 years younger to understand and, therefore, the denial of these feelings in the aged is a potential problem. A paraprofessional may have to work with the sexual acting out of a disturbed elderly patient or counsel and advise an elderly couple in this area. As one paraprofessional put it: "Clients often are sexually preoccupied!"

The gender and ethnic background of clients are important to keep in mind. In one instance, a white male paraprofessional was assigned to a retirement community in which 85% of the residents were black and female. He had little success working with this group. Much greater progress toward helping these clients was achieved when a black, female paraprofessional was assigned to this same area.

Volunteers are occasionally used to work with the elderly. If they are college students, their lack of available time and commitment is a problem. They have to be trained, and often they work for only one school quarter of 10 weeks. An alternative to using students is to use elderly people from the community who express interest in being volunteers. However, they sometimes have trouble working with the aging program because of the fear that they will face similar problems in their own future.

A major difficulty for the paraprofessional staff is the relatively low potential of their clients. These people are old, poor, often seriously disturbed, and alone. Help is remedial and ameliorative, and expectations have to be limited. While this realistic attitude is necessary, it still does not protect against the emotional involvement and disappointment at not achieving more. The paraprofessionals rely upon each other and the professional staff members for support and assistance in working through the often difficult feelings that their task engenders.

Use of Paraprofessionals

The paraprofessional mental health technicians spend the majority of their time out in the community. They are often called by a family member, a friend, or a neighbor to assist with an elderly person in a state of crisis. The client might be acting strangely; not taking care of personal needs such as food, hygiene, or physical health; afraid to leave a particular room; or too depressed to get out of bed. Fear is considered by the aging program staff to be the single biggest problem of the elderly.

The paraprofessional makes the initial evaluation of the client's need. They may have to get through the client's initial defenses in order to work with the client and gain the individual's trust. One approach at Hillsborough is for the paraprofessional to knock on a prospective client's door and say, "We hear you have a problem. We are from the aging program and would like to help you." The paraprofessionals downplay the "mental health" aspect of their role. Elderly clients often fear being taken away to a hospital. The center staff feel that a program working with older people must be careful in its selection of a name and should try to avoid the term "mental health" in the title of the program.

The paraprofessionals try to establish personal relationships with their clients. They do more physical touching than is done in professional therapeutic relationships. They are quick to state that most of their clients need a "friend" rather than a therapist. The clients, in turn, want to know about the paraprofessionals' lives. They think of them as sons or daughters. A paraprofessional said of the aging program, "We fill a need. If we didn't do these things, no one would."

The paraprofessionals work on practical matters such as helping their clients balance checkbooks, make shopping lists, or write letters. They go with them to get eyeglasses, hearing aids, or food stamps; they teach them proper nutrition or how to request homemaker services. They may read newspapers to clients, discuss current events, draw pictures, or get them to sing childhood or ethnic songs.

The staff members of the aging program feel that the first and most important accomplishment is to gain the trust of the client. Many clients, no matter how dire their circumstances, are loath to accept help. If they can be persuaded to talk about themselves, a bridge can be built. The paraprofessionals' role is to "try and see where they're coming from and why they're now like this." They feel it is important to work on the here and now—to dwell on the past brings out feelings of sorrow, remorse, and a sense of loss to many elderly clients. To deal with more than the immediate future may lead to feelings of hopelessness. Focusing on the present and on daily activities offers the most realistic and positive method of broadening the client's area of interpersonal encounter.

In this regard, one example stands out in its simplicity, realism, and awareness. The client was described as very old, very much alone, living in a trailer in the dark, and afraid to leave even to buy groceries. The paraprofessional suggested that the woman plant a flower garden and offered to help. While it was probably easier said than done, the effect was to move this lonely recluse out of her trailer and into the sunshine and to provide some meaning and purpose to her life. The garden was the first step in a series of efforts to get the client to buy herself food, get medical attention, and begin once more to care for herself.

Recruitment

The aging program does not actively recruit its paraprofessional staff. There are enough unsolicited applicants to fill the vacancies that arise. Only one of the paraprofessionals did not have a B.A. degree when starting the job. However, she had an A.A. degree in human service work and had served her internship at the center. Many college-educated people apply for the jobs, so the staff members feel no need to seek less formally educated people. The staff feel they have been much more successful when they have brought new people into the program, rather than when people have been transferred into the program from other parts of the mental health center. A number of the staff members interview applicants along with the director, although the final decision remains the responsibility of the director. The choice of a new staff member is certainly based on perceived competence, but it is clear that another important selection factor is compatibility—the ability to fit in or get along with the other staff members. This emphasis on compatibility in selecting new staff might be called a fraternity system.

The method of selecting staff members appears to be very crucial to a project's success. The advantage of the fraternity system may lie in its ability to produce a supportive atmosphere in which the employee can return for encouragement and support. This is important after the often frustrating and emotionally draining work of providing mental health services to the aging. One of the outstanding characteristics of the aging project is its esprit de corps and sense of mutual support. This mood is not created solely by selection procedures, but group involvement in the selection is most important. A possible disadvantage of the fraternity system for staff selection is that it could result in a rather homogeneous staff, with less variation in age, race, background, and style than might be desired.

Other qualities that the staff look for in a prospective member are flexibility, warmth, a desire to learn, and a sincere interest in and concern for older people. One paraprofessional stressed that people who are "too sensitive" should not be hired because of the inherent frustrations of the work. The staff members, indeed, often must face the death, suicide, and decline of clients for whom they had fond feelings.

Training

The aging program trains its new staff members by apprenticing them to more experienced staff members. There is little pre-service training; paraprofessionals are put into the field almost immediately. However, it is not merely a "sink or swim" situation because each paraprofessional has a great deal of support and supervision available from the more experienced paraprofessionals, as well as from the professional staff. There are in-service training sessions offered monthly by the center and by the aging program itself. These in-service sessions are not part of a planned curriculum. Rather, they tend to cover a variety of topics which are thought to be relevant and of interest. Such topics include reality orientation, drugs and the aging, chronic brain syndrome, transactional analysis, community resources, psychodrama, death and dying, and so on. While the staff members mention certain in-service sessions as having been helpful, it appears that they learn the most from their supervisory sessions with the project psychiatrist.

A small library of materials on aging has been set up in the director's office, and the staff psychiatrist lends articles or books to paraprofessionals who are curious about specific issues, but the emphasis is not on formal, academic training. There appear to be two reasons for this approach. First, the staff feel that the best learning comes from staff discussions about their direct experiences with clients; and second, the staff feel that there is very little printed material on aging that is useful in a practical way.

Supervision

Each of the five paraprofessionals in the aging program has access to the services of the staff psychiatrist for one hour a week. These five hours a week represent a relatively substantial investment by the project, but all the staff members feel it is well justified. The staff members may use their time with the psychiatrist in the way they feel is most useful. At present, the paraprofessionals usually bring in current clients, and the paraprofessionals and the psychiatrist develop a treatment plan relevant to the specific case. At other times, the psychiatrist and the paraprofessional might spend the time talking about mental health in general, the problems in aging, or some therapeutic technique. Still again, there are times when the paraprofessionals discuss a specific professional or even personal problem with him. At Hillsborough, the psychiatrist enjoys this supervision and also enjoys his relationships with the paraprofessionals, and they unanimously find him helpful. This informal style of supervision might not work in a setting where the psychiatrist is less interested in the staff members or less gifted in teaching, or where the relations between the paraprofessionals and the supervisor are poor. At the aging program, however, this method seems to work very well.

This availability of professional staff members to paraprofessionals for informal supervision is a striking feature of the aging program. As one paraprofessional put it, "You don't feel like you are imposing." In understaffed, crisis-oriented mental health programs, staff members often feel reluctant, even guilty, about seeking out the assistance, and taking up the time, of the supervisor. In addition, the supervisors are sometimes resentful of the time they must devote to supervision rather than to providing direct services.

The director of the aging project also supervises the paraprofessionals work. She spends an average of 15 hours per week in this capacity. To keep informed about the clients, she reads the case reports that the paraprofessionals write. She also does personnel reviews annually, and raises are based on these reviews. The director tends to share many of her administrative problems with the staff. She discusses policy questions with them. This procedure not only keeps the staff informed but gives the director support in her role.

Mobility

Upward job mobility for the paraprofessionals in the aging program is very limited. Although the center has a job descriptions for mental health technicians (paraprofessionals) which span four different salary levels, all the paraprofessionals were hired at Level 2 ($6,526 a year), and there was only one Level 4 slot ($8,332) for a mental health technician in the entire center, which was already filled. Thus, there is opportunity for paraprofessional upward mobility in theory, but functionally there is only one level in the hierarchy.

Education

While the Hillsborough Community Mental Health Center believes that training for paraprofessionals is valuable, the in-service training offered by the center and the aging program is not accredited by a college, nor does it lead to a promotion. There is support for those paraprofessionals who choose to continue their education, but the center has no formal policy for aiding in this endeavor. Two of the paraprofessionals originally hired have left the aging program to go back to school, one in social work and the other in geriatrics.

Status and Morale

The professional and paraprofessional staff members get along together extremely well. They often eat together, share leisure time, and generally view each other as friends as well as colleagues. The substantially higher salaries earned by the professional staff, particularly by the occupational therapist and the recreational therapist who have no more college education than most of the paraprofessionals, cause some resentment and engender feelings of guilt on the part of these professional staff members. Basically, however, the paraprofessional staff members feel appreciated and respected by the professional staff. The psychiatrist, for example, in his case notes always refers to a client as "belonging" to a specific paraprofessional.

Because of the current structure of third-party payments (that is, health insurance reimbursements), the cost of a service offered by a paraprofessional cannot be reimbursed, while the same service offered by a psychiatrist can be. There is concern about the effect of third-party payment rules on the staffing patterns of programs at the Hillsborough Community Mental Health Center. If such policies continue and such payments eventually become the financial mainstay of the center, then there will necessarily be a dramatic decrease in the use of paraprofessionals.

Another problem paraprofessionals experience is difficulty in dealing with staff members from other agencies who see the paraprofessionals as lacking authority. For example, the staff members at a state hospital tend not to respond to the request of the paraprofessional in charge of a project, but a request appears to carry more weight when a social worker makes it. On the other hand, the paraprofessional staff members feel that they are able to establish meaningful relationships more quickly with a client because the client does not have to break through an aura of professionalism.

Evaluation

The aging program has a half-time evaluator who is paid out of special center funds. Thus, the sizable amount of evaluation done within this program is probably atypical. The quality of its evaluation component is also probably atypical. Speculation about *why* the evaluation component of the aging program was so well received by the staff and so well integrated into the program might assist other programs to improve their evaluations.

First, the evaluator was hired at the beginning of the program. This meant that the staff members saw the gathering of data as part of their job when they were hired. It was not seen as something added onto an already busy schedule. Furthermore, the evaluator gets along well with the staff members. The staff members' acceptance of him as a person facilitated their acceptance of him as an evaluator. The evaluator makes an effort to be reasonable in his demands for information; he listens to the concerns of the staff members and takes their criticisms seriously. For example, one evaluation instrument required staff members to ask nursing home patients about their perceptions of the future. This specific question upset a number of patients and was finally dropped because it was not seen as important enough to justify upsetting clients.

The evaluator suggests that evaluation instruments be brief, as aging clients often have short attention spans. He stresses the need to train the staff who administer the questionnaires because the quality of the data gathered by untrained staff may be so poor as to be invalid.

Finally, the evaluator shares his findings with the paraprofessional staff. He lets them know what the scores mean. Staff members like being able to find out their success in certain areas, and they pride themselves on the fact that the evaluator's data confirm their gut feelings that clients do improve.

In Conclusion

As the proportion of our population over 55 years of age increases, mental health centers will have to provide services geared to the special needs of this population. Their problems are complex and include social and physical isolation, poverty, poor health, inadequate transportation, and lack of meaningful activities and recreation. These problems may create or exacerbate mental health problems for the aged.

Paraprofessionals are ideally suited to be part of the treatment team working with older clients. They can go into the community to serve clients who find it difficult or impossible to come to centers or to satellite clinics. They can provide friendship and practical assistance to lonely people facing practical problems. The Hillsborough Community Mental Health Center's aging program has demonstrated that well-chosen, well-trained, and well-supervised paraprofessionals can provide consultation and training to other agencies that have contact with older clients, as well as serve as liaisons between these agencies and the center. Working closely with the professional staff, paraprofessionals can provide a wide variety of services to meet the needs of older citizens.

Chapter 3

ALCOHOL ABUSE SERVICES

INTRODUCTION

Description of the Service Area

The provision of alcohol services has historically been an area that has been neglected by mental health professionals. "Repeated surveys of professional agencies and professional attitudes indicate that there is a general negativistic attitude toward alcoholics, that generic service agencies ignore or screen out alcoholics, much less make measured efforts to make their services available to them, and that professionals both avoid choosing services to alcoholics as a professional option and avoid those who seek services in their agencies."[1]

The original result of these attitudes was that the treatment of alcoholics was primarily the domain of volunteers and paraprofessionals. At present, the field is still poorly organized, with a limited number of relevant training possibilities available at the paraprofessional level. Few professionals choose to specialize in the treatment of persons with alcohol abuse problems, when this option is available, and certainly no consensus in theory or philosophy exists to guide any group of practitioners in a concerted effort.

[1]As quoted in Pattison, E. M., M.D. A differential view of manpower resources. In Staub, E. E. & Kent, L. M. (Eds.), *The paraprofessional in the treatment of alcoholism.* Springfield, Ill.: Bannerstone House, 1973.

National Institute of Mental Health guidelines state that a federally funded community mental health center must provide alcohol abuse service programs except when there is documented evidence that such need does not exist in a catchment area, or where such need is currently being met by other social service agencies.

The center should designate at least one staff member as administratively responsible for implementation of alcohol abuse services, and should in addition assign multidisciplinary professionals at least part time to this task.

The program should make all needed services of the center available to alcohol clients. These would include, for example, outpatient, inpatient, partial hospitalization, and emergency services. Detoxification services must also be arranged. The alcohol program should interface with consultation and education services, and should have planned preventive strategies. Liaison and coordination with relevant community social and rehabilitative agencies should be accomplished.

Selection of the Site Visited

The selection of the site for an effective model of alcohol services was the result of a nationwide search. All regional Department of Health, Education, and Welfare (HEW) offices were contacted and their opinions solicited. A computer search was undertaken through the National Institute of Alcohol Abuse and Alcoholism (NIAAA), seeking programs that satisfied our criteria regarding good use of paraprofessionals to provide effective services. Eventually, more than 30 different programs were recommended for further investigation. After a preliminary screening of the original list, extensive telephone interviews were conducted with administrative personnel from centers and independent programs in Florida, Colorado, California, Utah, Minnesota, Texas, Massachusetts, Hawaii, and Arizona.

One result of these interviews was a profile of similarities between programs in this area. All such programs consider regular training in alcohol-related issues and treatment alternatives essential for alcohol staff members. A particular emphasis is placed on knowing the various underlying disorders that may be masked by alcohol usage.

Outreach programs are emphasized as the modality necessary to have an impact on problem drinkers. This direct service task is often complemented by prevention efforts. In addition to prevention work with individuals, project staff tend to work with social service agencies to help them improve and coordinate their efforts towards people with alcohol problems. Good working relationships are reported with these related agencies.

Accreditation of alcohol programs is a topic that concerns each administrator. Most centers contacted state that they have received accreditation or are prepared for it, and have requested the joint commission to visit the site. Accreditation is viewed as important for reasons of program status, prestige, and legitimacy. Financial benefits in terms of third party payments, however, are viewed with a certain skepticism.

The alcohol component of each center is funded by at least one, and usually by a number of special grants. This funding is specific for alcohol-related service delivery and is separate and distinct from other, more general funding such as staffing or construction grants. Salaries for alcohol counselors seem to be generally better than for paraprofessionals working in other service areas.

Centers often report relationships with nearby universities and colleges that involve their alcohol staff. Students from the schools do internships or fieldwork under the supervision of the paraprofessional alcohol staff members, who also teach courses or appear as guest speakers in classes. In addition, paraprofessionals frequently take courses and receive field credit for work towards degrees.

The Permian Basin Centers for Mental Health and Mental Retardation located in Midland, Texas, were initially recommended by the Department of Health, Education, and Welfare regional office in Dallas for offering an effective alcohol services program. It was selected as a site because it embodied our two primary criteria, good service delivery and good use of paraprofessionals.

The delivery of alcohol services at Midland is provided by a multiracial, bilingual staff, who place a strong emphasis on outreach, prevention, and community involvement. The staff members offer a good model of complementary paraprofessional-professional relationships. Finally, the center shows a strong commitment to paraprofessionals' personal growth, development, and in-center mobility, including an emphasis on continual ongoing training.

PERMIAN BASIN CENTERS FOR MENTAL HEALTH AND MENTAL RETARDATION: A CASE STUDY IN ALCOHOL SERVICES*

South of the Texas Panhandle, midway between El Paso and Dallas/Fort Worth, is an area known as the Permian Basin. With its headquarters and clinic in Midland and another clinic located in the neighboring town of Odessa, the Permian Basin Centers for Mental Health and Mental Retardation provide services for a catchment population of 160,000. The service delivery system is characterized by active community involvement, a paraprofessional director,

*Contact: Permian Basin Centers for Mental Health and Mental Retardation
        3701 North Big Springs
        Midland, Texas   79701
        915/683-5591
        Attention: Robert Dickson, Center Director
                Joe Glass, Program Director

a "business model" organization, a staff that is 80% paraprofessional, and a philosophy that emphasizes community and service.

Services to alcoholics are provided by six paraprofessionals who are under the direct supervision of three professional staff members. Four of the paraprofessionals are alcoholism counselors, and two community service aides were recently hired as assistant alcoholism counselors. The six counselors are not part of a separate program but rather are considered to be staff members of the outpatient programs. Two counselors and one assistant counselor work out of the Odessa clinic, and two counselors and one assistant counselor work out of the Midland offices. In addition, the center has a contract with Park Place, a nonmedical detoxification facility, where alcoholics can dry out.

The Permian Basin center provides a wide range of alcohol services. These include crisis intervention, individual counseling and group therapy, and a large amount of community work. Outreach efforts aimed at individuals and families have been augmented by the two assistant alcohol counselors. One specializes in working with the county's black population (7%); the other works with the Chicano population (12%).

The alcohol counselors do consultation with various public agencies such as schools, social agencies, and the law enforcement network. They have established a number of useful liaisons to coordinate the work of those agencies involved with alcoholics. There is also an effort to gain the cooperation of private industry in dealing with employees who have drinking problems.

Background

Prior to 1950, the area surrounding Midland was primarily ranching and farm land. The discovery of oil has had a major impact on the people who live here. Construction of various industry headquarters in the downtown section, a rapidly expanding network of suburban homesites surrounding the city, and all of the work connected with oil recovery have created a rapidly expanding economy.

As is typical in oil towns, the image of a "real man" is often perceived to be a capacity for "hard working" and "hard drinking." Extremely high levels of alcohol consumption are tolerated and even expected. As one citizen puts it: "More business deals are carried on at the 007 Club [a local bar] than at the Wilco building."

The people in the Midland area who are concerned with mental health feel that this attitude towards alcohol and the ensuing number of alcoholic casualties make alcohol the major mental health problem in the area. Robert Dickson, the director of the Permian Basin center, has been involved with this problem, particularly as an alcoholism counselor, since 1967. Prior to developing the center, he was a successful businessman. His personal experience with alcohol made him want to help others with similar problems. He went through a counselor training program and worked as a paraprofessional volunteer in the alcoholism program of a state hospital.

Robert Dickson sets the general tone of the center, which is positive and open. The staff members talk about him with respect, admiration, and warmth. He is not perceived as a distant power figure but rather as a man to whom they can talk, as someone who will understand. He also is close to his staff members. He knows what they are doing, if they are having problems, who is going to school, and who has an idea that might improve the centers' programs. He personally interviewed each person before they were hired and this probably has something to do with the close relationships. Staff members feel that he is "willing to put his neck on the line and take the heat when paraprofessionals are questioned."

The Midland area had a very limited number of social services available in the late 1960s. The traditional conservative viewpoint towards government agencies' interfering with individual lives was partially responsible for this. Services for alcoholics, for example, were limited to Alcoholics Anonymous and to the state hospital. Both of these programs imposed severe restrictions on who could be helped and in what manner. In addition, the hospital had no follow-up, partial care, or counseling services for its clients.

It was a political decision to construct a school for the mentally retarded in a different community that finally mobilized concerned citizens to do something about the social service needs of Midland. Robert Dickson, along with citizens from a wide variety of occupations and roles, began a two-year planning effort aimed at the development of a mental health and mental retardation center.

A board of trustees established fact-finding committees composed of citizens and personnel from existing agencies. Their goal was to identify the community needs that were not being met by ongoing efforts. The concerned citizens generated interest by focusing on the plight of the community's mentally retarded children. The group took this approach because, as one source put it: "Nobody wants to talk to you about alcoholics or crazy people."

Robert Dickson was asked to be the director of the new center. He convinced the board that the mental health center should be modeled after a business organization. He felt that the combination of good business sense with caring and concern for individuals would result in a successful mental health center.

Robert Dickson planned for the mental health center staffing needs with a consultant who is a psychologist. The consultant advised that Ph.D. psychologists were unnecessary, and that M.A. level psychologists could provide satisfactory professional services. In Texas, psychologists with masters degrees are licensed as psychological associates. The center has not hired a single Ph.D psychologist, and psychiatrists are used at the center solely on a consulting basis. Most services are provided by paraprofessionals, who receive regular training and supervision by the professionals.

The philosophy of the center is simply stated by Dickson: "Timely and effective help for those hurting, delivered in an appropriate manner at the least practical cost." The old fashioned businessman's view is encouraged—that is, satisfy the customer. "We feel that folks here should be responsive to the needs of the community. We are a service organization. We should be prepared to deal at midnight with a crisis."

The center began with a staff of two B.A. level caseworkers, two M.A. psychologists, and a consulting psychiatrist. At present, it has grown to 110 staff members, 81 of whom have less than a master's degree. The budget is $1,700,000 annually.

The treatment of alcoholics was an important priority for the Midland center. In 1973, funds were obtained from the Texas Commission on Alcoholism (TCA) to hire four alcohol counselors. They were all experienced, previously trained individuals who had dealt with the problem personally, either themselves or with their families.

A physician at the state hospital, concerned about the lengthy waiting list for admission to the alcohol ward and the number of people turned away for various reasons, worked with the center to develop Park Place, a residential nonmedical detoxification unit. The state hospital pays for 100% of the staff salaries for this unit. It was developed as a separate organization, working under contract to the mental health center. Park Place receives technical assistance from the Permian Basin alcohol counselors.

In the fall of 1976, the TCA again provided funds that enabled the center to hire two assistant alcoholism counselors to operate a neighborhood alcohol program. This type of outreach work is also done by the center's paraprofessional staff members who are community service aides. The particular focus of the assistant alcohol counselors is the development of relationships between the center and minority communities to create awareness of the services available to those persons who have drinking problems.

Program Organization and Services

At the Permian center, the staff members of the alcohol service try to be realistic about whom they can help. The upper middle class drinker is not the focus of their efforts. The Permian Basin community does not view heavy drinking as a problem, and may, in fact, glorify it. The typical white-collar drinker may maintain a successful outward appearance, get his work done, have adequate social relations, and be a pillar of the community. He may maintain this image until his drinking problem results in a personal catastrophe, for example, killing himself while driving drunk, having a heart attack, or getting cirrhosis of the liver. If he does seek help, it will usually be in a different town, one where he is not known. Joe Glass, the center's program director, notes that a shift in cultural attitude is needed in order to change community attitudes towards drinking.

In the Permian Basin center, the blue-collar worker and the unemployed, marginal drinker are typically the people who receive treatment. Such people have less social status to lose; having a problem has less of a stigma attached to it, and receiving the attention of a social service agency is somewhat more acceptable. The average alcohol-related client at the Permian Basin center is male (86%), between the ages of 21 and 64 (95%), and Caucasian (88%), with an income of less than $50 a week.

The paraprofessional alcohol counselors provide a variety of services for their clients. These include traditional outpatient modalities such as diagnosis, individual and family counseling, and group therapy. Crisis intervention, client advocacy with social agencies, and assistance finding work are other common tasks.

The challenge of getting problem drinkers to come to the center and ask for help has led to a heavy emphasis on outreach work. The paraprofessional alcohol counselors are particularly effective here because of their intimate knowledge of the alcoholics' habits and habitats.

The Park Place facility serves as an important stepping stone to treatment. It is located a mile from the center in an aging Spanish-style motel. It attracts alcoholics who need drying out. The facility is shabby and run down. A center administrator said jokingly, "The place has a sobering effect on the alcoholic. He wakes up, looks around and asks, 'How in the hell did I end up here?' " Nonetheless, because long sought after funding has become available, two new detoxification facilities are presently being constructed by the center.

Park Place is a short-term residential facility. Winos, hoboes, and others seriously disabled by drinking can stay there, dry out, get fed, receive counseling, and get connected with employment training agencies. The use of nonmedical settings such as Park Place versus medically-oriented drying out facilities is a controversial question in the alcohol field. The decision to use a nonmedical facility originally was made because it costs less to run than a facility that employs medical doctors. In addition, the experience of staff members led them to believe that the effectiveness of a nonmedical setting is increased because it does not use doctors. Said a Permian Basin staff member: "The medical approach gives the alcoholic an out. He does not have to take responsibility for his problem because it is a disease that the doctor will cure."

The Park Place staff is usually recruited from the center's "alcoholic" clientele. Some work as volunteers for a time. Staff members are selected from those volunteers who appear to be capable workers. Training of these staff members and their daily supervision is the responsibility of one of the center's alcohol counselors. A psychologist (M.A. level) has overall responsibility for the alcohol staff members. The staff is trained particularly to identify those clients who require attention. Since this is a nonmedical facility, any case suspected of requiring a physician's attention must be transferred to a hospital.

Once a client is dried out, a case conference is held with the Park Place staff members, the center staff members, and the client to determine a treatment plan. The client's view of his problems is solicited. Various alternatives are outlined. These include individual counseling, group therapy, vocational rehabilitation, and psychological testing.

While this program does not run along traditional Alcoholics Anonymous (A.A.) lines, much of what the counselors do is influenced by the A.A. approach. However, certain A.A. rules, such as limitations on eligibility for treatment or expulsion from the program of clients who have drinking bouts, are not imposed. The alcohol counselors have developed relationships with local agencies such as the family service agencies and law enforcement officers at the jails to get them to refer those people who have alcohol problems. A local judge gives alcoholics the choice between jail or treatment. The police request the alcohol counselors' assistance in dealing with families in a crisis situation over a problem drinker.

In general, the alcohol counselor goes wherever there are people with drinking problems. The counselors seek to educate these people concerning the alternatives open to them. If the people do not wish to go to the center for treatment, then treatment takes place where they are. Problem drinkers are counseled in private homes, neighborhood bars, jails, and on the street, as well as at the hospitals.

The success of the alcohol program is determined by several outcome measurements. The program has cut the admissions to the state hospital alcohol ward by two-thirds in the last two years. In 1974, the rate was 1.43 admissions per 1,000 population. In 1976, this had decreased to 0.37 per 1,000. The cost of service to those treated by the center is considerably below the hospital cost. The average cost for detoxification at Park Place is $23.40 per contact. The state hospital cost is estimated at $56 to $57 per day. For the fiscal year 1975–76, 502 clients received 24-hour care and 608 received outpatient counseling.

Park Place clients are evaluated by a method known as Goal Attainment Scoring[2] (GAS). A three month follow-up interview is attempted to determine the effectiveness of treatment. This is a difficult undertaking, since it is a transient population that primarily makes use of the facility. For the first three quarters of 1976, 290 clients completed an intake GAS. Three months after treatment, 24% of these (70) were able to be contacted. Follow-up scores averaged 55.74 (s.d. 16.06) compared to an intake mean of 25.14 (s.d. 4.33). This points to substantial changes in clients' behavior as viewed by themselves and their counselors.

An Additional Note on the Organization of Alcohol Services.   The problem of identification with the team (alcohol services) versus identification with the organization (the center) was recently faced and handled by the Permian Basin administration. The alcohol counselors had been working as a

[2]Kirezuk, Thomas J., & Sherman, Robert E. Goal Attainment Scoring: A general method for evaluating comprehensive community mental health programs. *Community Mental Health Journal,* 1968, *4,* 443–453.

unit out of the Midland office. They developed close interpersonal relationships based on mutual support in handling a difficult task. The administration felt that the unit was becoming too much of a clique.

The responsibilities of the alcohol counselors require a great deal of liaison and communication with all other members of the center's staff. In order to ensure continuity of care, alcohol clients may require an alcohol counselor as the primary treatment contact, but often can make use of psychological testing, day care treatment, psychotherapy, or other additional services. It was the administration's opinion that by identifying too strongly with a subgroup, the alcohol staff member has more difficulty in working well with other units, to the detriment of client care.

The decision was made to divide the supervision of the counselors in the Midland outpatient treatment unit. The alcoholism counselors are required to report to different supervisors in order to structure them into more significant contact with other staff members. The decision was made with the view that it was for the good of the overall functioning of the center.

Use of Paraprofessionals

The primary reason for using paraprofessional staff members at the Permian Basin center is cost. Paraprofessional workers cost less per unit of service than do professional staff members. Robert Dickson believes that, based on his experience with paraprofessionals who have thorough training and ongoing supervision, they can accomplish the service delivery goals of the center.

Yet at the same time Dickson believes that in no way is the cheaper service second-class service. "If I had no cost restrictions, I would hire the same people who now work for me. They do the job—that's what's necessary." Thus, the original impetus to hire paraprofessional staff, i.e., lower cost, has been superseded by the awareness that their unique skills and abilities are well suited to the tasks at a community mental health center.

The conservative Texas population's inherent distrust of government agencies makes it necessary for mental health workers to go out into the community and educate the people regarding the services available. This is not a traditional professional role. Many professionals are uncomfortable doing anything that might be interpreted as soliciting clients. Thus, the paraprofessional workers' lack of preconceived notions about their roles allows them to undertake the requirements of this assigned task more comfortably.

In the specific area of alcohol services, everyone interviewed at the center agreed that the paraprofessional counselor is best able to work as the primary treatment coordinator for the alcoholic client. Formal education aside, there is no substitute for the experience of having been an alcoholic, or having lived with one.

The center staff members believe that the recovered alcoholic who is a counselor will become a positive role model for the alcoholic struggling with his problem. The client will have continued proof that someone with a similar plight was successful in overcoming it. This provides hope for the alcoholic.

Often, in community mental health centers, professional staff members do not like to treat alcoholics. They do not feel that the usual psychotherapy techniques, for example, have much impact. The professional staff members at the Permian Basin center are pleased that the paraprofessional alcohol counselors are available to handle these clients. Having "been there themselves," the counselors know how to confront the myriad of "games" that are the alcoholics' typical way of relating to themselves and others.

What Paraprofessionals Do

The alcohol counselors provide all direct and indirect services to alcohol clients. They each carry 20 to 30 open cases. They are supervised by three professionals, two social workers and an M.A. psychologist. They are responsible for the outpatient services to clients with alcohol problems. After a client arrives, the counselor does an intake history/background and then makes a diagnosis. The counselors are trained to recognize the types of cases that will require additional assistance. For example, clients with medical problems are immediately referred to a physician or a hospital. In addition, some clients use alcohol to deal with severe psychological problems such as schizophrenia. The training sessions in diagnosis and assessment help the counselors to recognize these underlying disorders, and such clients are then referred to professional staff.

The counselors do not see themselves as doing psychotherapy. They do counseling in such areas as value clarification, helping the clients to see the choices they have and to make decisions. The counselors provide information, aiding clients to see how they are harming themselves and how they might help themselves. They run groups and focus on getting the clients to discuss their problems, feelings, and hopes with each other.

The counselors work with the families of clients, and if possible with their clients' employers. They assist these other important people in the alcoholic's life to understand the nature of the alcohol problem and to suggest types of support that the client needs in order to overcome problems. They do follow-up visits to the client's home for up to two years after the client is discharged from treatment.

Crisis work is a normal part of the job. Calls can come in at any hour. The police recognize the skills of the counselors in working with "drunks" who are creating a problem in the community. One counselor makes a point, as he travels around the community, of giving out his phone number and letting people know he is available.

The counselors work in conjunction with the state hospital and the local Veterans Administration (V.A.) hospital. They meet with alcohol ward clients who are preparing for discharge. They suggest outpatient treatment plans, talk to families, seek out employment opportunities, or contact the state vocational rehabilitation staff. Prevention talks are part of the counselors' responsibility. They work with the local schools to create an awareness of the problems of alcohol and to raise issues for discussion by the children. They have tried, with marginal success, to introduce prevention programs into private industry.

The assistant alcohol counselors were hired with the specific aim of developing neighborhood alcohol programs in the minority communities. Their responsibilities with this population are similar to those of the alcohol counselors. They carry ongoing client case loads; run therapy groups; work in the field visiting bars, schools, homes, churches, and other places where people congregate; do information and education talks; and make referrals to the center or the hospitals when necessary.

Recruitment

Finding qualified people is difficult in the Permian Basin area. It is not a major urban center, and people interested in working in a social service organization do not often come to town. Those who do come are interested in oil and money. If qualified people can be located, the center prefers to recruit staff members from the community it serves.

Considering the outreach focus of the center, knowledge of the area is considered very useful. A primary source of recruitment is from within the center's own ranks. Volunteers serve as a source of workers. Personnel who are capable are promoted to better jobs whenever possible. The model for this action is Robert Dickson, the center's director, who entered the field as a volunteer.

When in-house staff members are not available for a position then the center advertises widely. In particular, the state hospital is a source for experienced personnel.

Selection

The selection process involves three lengthy interviews. First, the prospective employee is interviewed by the supervisor who will have primary responsibility for the applicant's activities. Then either Joe Glass, the center's program director, or Robert Dickson interviews the applicant. Finally, the applicant is interviewed by the board of trustees. This procedure is followed for all positions. The qualifications of the applicant are discussed with the people they will work with and their reactions are sought. The final decision is made by the board of trustees. All these steps in the hiring procedure result in a high level of awareness on the part of the administrative personnel regarding the employees of the center.

Except in the case of specific grants, there are no educational degree requirements that the Permian Basin centers have to meet in hiring. They do not have a state or county personnel system to act as an external constraint on their hiring. Their practice is to define the job and determine the talents, skills, and capabilities that a person must have to fill the role successfully. In the case of alcohol counselors, several such requirements have been determined. With the exception of one assistant counselor, all counselors are middle-aged persons. This is not a specific requirement, but the necessary life experience generally precludes young counselors. Although it is not an absolute requirement, personal experience with alcoholism is an important consideration. All counselors, with the exception of one assistant counselor, have been alcoholics or have had an alcoholic in their immediate family. In the case of recovered alcoholics, two years of continual sobriety is the minimum requirement. Prior experience and training in counseling methods are considered essential to providing alcohol services. All counselors had worked previously as counselors, usually in a volunteer capacity. Two counselors had gone through extensive programs offered by other organizations with the express aim of training alcohol counselors.

The staff members believe that it is important for a counselor to have certain personal characteristics. The counselor should be "a worker, a hustler, someone who cares about people." The job requires someone who can work independently in the community, yet be able to coordinate efforts with other members of the team and with other programs in the centers. This person has to be able to speak "the language of the streets," as well as work effectively with professionals in agencies, such as judges, police, probation officers, school principals, teachers, and doctors. This person should feel a sense of mission so that a midnight crisis call is dealt with at midnight—the job is more than an 8:00 to 5:00 commitment.

Three counselors are female and three are male. The assistant alcohol counselors, a Mexican-American woman and a black man, were hired specifically to work with the area's ethnic and minority populations. They work closely with the other alcohol counselors. This need had been recognized for some time, but had to wait until necessary funding became available. The black man is the exception to most of the stated experiential requirements. He is in his twenties, is not an alcoholic, nor is he related to an alcoholic. He had no previous volunteer alcoholism counselor experience, but had past experience in working with youth and those with drug problems. He is working as an alcohol counselor presently to help black persons with alcohol problems, and to educate himself further about the challenge of this aspect of helping others.

Training

Ongoing training at the Permian Basin center is considered to be of primary importance to effective service delivery. According to Robert Dickson: "People should keep up with current thinking and new ideas." All training is focused on the development of skills in a particular area related to the staff member's task performance.

Once a week, an in-service training session is held. This might focus on diagnostic and assessment skills, or perhaps on a specific counseling approach such as transactional analysis or Gestalt therapy. Any staff member who has a specific area of interest will present it at a training session. Occasionally, paraprofessional workers are sent out of state to attend workshops or conferences. These staff members then present what they have learned at the training session to the rest of the center staff workers.

A case conference is held once a week with a consulting psychiatrist. Ongoing cases that the counselors feel they need help in evaluating are presented and discussed. Diagnoses are made and treatment approaches are suggested. Whenever there has been a sizable staff turnover the psychiatrist will present basic useful medical information about medications or nosology (disease classifications).

The state hospital has a monthly conference attended by the alcohol counselors. Persons of nationally recognized importance give presentations and workshops.

Much training goes on informally. "Our training consists of doing it," said one counselor. The close working relationships ensure that skills sharing and problem solving go on continually. A supervisor mentioned that a center needs a core group of experienced paraprofessionals who can take new employees "under the wing" for an initial on-the-job training period.

There is now an additional reason for the alcohol counselors to get training. The Texas Association of Alcoholism Counselors (P.O. Box 221, Austin, Texas 78767) has recently completed development of a peer certification system for alcohol counselors. The purpose of this certification is twofold: to control the evaluation of practitioners, assuring counselor qualifications at the statewide level; and to provide the individual practitioner with a credential which certifies his/her professional competency.

In addition to prior experience as an alcohol counselor, certification is dependent upon 200 hours of continuing education in approved alcoholism counselor training courses. All of the Permian Basin alcohol counselors were interested in obtaining certification. However, since the system is new, they were not certain as to the benefits to be expected. They felt that there could be potential benefits in terms of status, mobility, and perhaps salary. The success of the system was thought to be related to how powerful the alcohol counselor organization became.

Supervision

The counselors receive both formal and informal supervision. They have at least two meetings each week to discuss ongoing cases with professional supervisors. Informal checking with each other on problems or new ideas is a commonplace occurrence, and formal peer level supervision groups are being planned.

Career Mobility

The alcohol counselors did not consider the issue of job mobility as relevant to them. They have come to their work in their middle years, and see it in terms of a mission rather than a job. They feel that their reward lies in the satisfaction of helping others who are undergoing the same problems they have faced. They do not want to take on other duties of a supervisory nature. One young assistant alcohol counselor does have plans to return to school to obtain a master's degree. Mobility within the center does not interest him as much as the opportunity his work offers him to gain experience in the field.

Education

While staff are encouraged to go to school, and a college degree is necessary for advancement to supervisory responsibilities, a college education for a staff member is not seen as the center's responsibility. If a person wishes to work towards a college degree, assistance is offered in terms of flexible scheduling of work assignments, or by being allowed to work half time. Paid time off is not offered.

A number of paraprofessionals have obtained master's degrees while working full time and have moved into higher positions. It is well recognized that the center would like to put its own people into these positions and thus there is an incentive to put out extra effort in terms of schooling. There is a college in the area that offers an accredited master's degree program with different behavioral science options. Field work credit for on-the-job experience is offered.

Status and Morale

The alcohol counselors feel that their work is appreciated. They know that what they do is essential to the center and that they are the only staff members capable of successfully accomplishing it. They work well together and with their professional supervisors. The professionals have learned through personal experience that the paraprofessional staff members handle their duties very competently. One supervisor reported that because of his background, which emphasized educational preparation, he felt that treatment could only be accomplished by a professionally trained person. His observation of the success of the alcohol counselors working in groups, handling crisis calls, and training volunteers, has caused him to reconsider his original viewpoint. It took him a while to come to this conclusion, but he now believes that the paraprofessionals provide a high quality of service.

The alcohol counselors have feelings common to most of the programs visited. They like their work and feel they are treated with respect; they have a great deal of individual autonomy; their work is essential to the center and difficult to accomplish. However, their salary is limited to a range below the level of personnel with formal education. The salary range for alcohol counselors is $10,512 to $13,248; for assistant counselors $7,560 to $9,528. The cause for complaint, in this case, does not seem to be the actual salary, but rather what the salary limitation means in terms of status and personal value. To the alcohol counselors, the message is that they will always be worth less than personnel who have more formal education.

Evaluation

Evaluation of alcohol counselors at the Permian Basin centers occurs informally on a weekly basis, when counselors present cases in staffing conferences, and also during case discussions with supervisors. Formal evaluation is made with the assistance of a comprehensive yearly evaluation report that rates counselors on such items as knowledge of work, quantity and quality of work, ability to learn new duties, initiative, cooperation, judgment, common sense, and record keeping. The report includes an open-ended narrative section. Supervisors prepare this form for each counselor, and discuss their opinions with their staff.

In Conclusion

The Permian Basin Centers for Mental Health and Mental Retardation offer a useful example of effective mental health service delivery, dictated by the needs of the community, and provided by paraprofessional and professional staff working together in a complementary relationship. The use of paraprofessionals in all service areas is a key factor in allowing the center to offer its innovative kinds of services to the largest number of persons seeking help. Further, through paraprofessional outreach activities, these services are offered to those who would otherwise be unaware of the help available.

By focusing on the delivery of alcohol services, we have provided an in-depth view of paraprofessional utilization that is representative of the center's overall commitment in this regard. The attention that the center's administration pays to careful selection, sound ongoing training, and regular supervision of the paraprofessional staff, as well as to personal concerns such as career mobility, status, and continuing education, should be considered as essential to the quality of services provided.

Chapter 4

CHILDREN'S SERVICES

INTRODUCTION

Description of the Service Area

Specialized services for children were first legally mandated by the 1975 Community Mental Health Center Amendments, although some federal funds supported relevant mental health center programs prior to that time. According to the National Institute of Mental Health guidelines, a children's program is required to provide a range of diagnostic, treatment, liaison, and follow-up services to children from birth to age 18. These services should be based on a community assessment of needs for (1) indirect (consultation and education) and preventive services, and (2) direct services. A children's program, furthermore, should include the full range of services offered through the center, appropriately oriented to the needs of children at different stages of development. For example, a therapeutic nursery may be the appropriate means for providing day care for younger children. The services should incorporate a variety of treatment modalities, be adapted to the needs of physically handicapped children, and, where relevant, be geared to the participation of the family. Satellite facilities and home visits should be provided for clients who cannot be served in the base facility of the mental health center.

Selection of the Site Visited

Seven children's programs were recommended as effective by Department of Health, Education, and Welfare regional offices, as well as by mental health professionals specializing in children's services. Most of these children's programs involve paraprofessionals in the provision of consultation and education services. About one-half of the programs involve paraprofessionals in day care services; about one-half involve paraprofessionals in outpatient services. Services in other program areas (e.g., emergency) may be available to children, but are usually offered through the other service units of the mental health center. The programs surveyed do not characteristically offer specialized services for children at different stages of development. Furthermore, the programs tend to offer most services at central locations rather than through home visits or satellite-based facilities. The services also tend to focus specifically on the child, rather than on the family as a treatment unit. However, a number of the programs do offer services designed to prevent the development of mental health problems in children.

Paraprofessionals perform a variety of direct and indirect functions within the mental health center as well as in homes, schools, and community-based facilities. While the paraprofessionals do provide consultation and education services to school teachers, they do not generally provide these services to mental health professionals. Generally, the children's programs employ from two to six full-time paraprofessionals. However, one program employs 25 paid paraprofessionals (five hours daily) in a partial hospitalization program. Another program employs 43 full-time paraprofessionals in partial hospitalization and inpatient programs. One of the centers provides an extensive federally funded training program to prepare paraprofessionals for work in children's programs.

The children's program of the Huntsville-Madison County Mental Health Center was highly recommended by the Department of Health, Education, and Welfare Regional Office in Atlanta as well as by the Southern Regional Education Board. The Huntsville Children's Program offers a well-designed array of services to both children and their families. The program offers these services through outpatient, day treatment, and consultation and education divisions. Paraprofessionals participate in all three service areas. In addition, the Huntsville program is unique among those children's programs surveyed in that it offers, in one setting, training of paraprofessionals to be assertive with their professional supervisors; ongoing feedback to paraprofessionals about their performance; systematic rewards to paraprofessionals (and professionals) for competence; encouragement of paraprofessional participation in research, with listing of paraprofessionals as authors of resulting publications; and assembling of valid data on the effectiveness of paraprofessionals.

Huntsville-Madison County Mental Health Center: A Case Study in Children's Services*

The Huntsville-Madison County Community Mental Health Center serves the 185,000 residents of Huntsville, Alabama and the surrounding region of Madison County. The center consists of three independently organized components: the Support Program, the Adult Program, and the Child and Parent Program. The Support Program is the administrative, evaluation, training, and research arm of the center. It is responsible for monitoring and compiling information supplied by the Adult Program and the Child and Parent Program, the two clinical arms of the center. This chapter focuses on the mental health services to children, adolescents, and families as delivered by the Child and Parent Program of the center.

The Child and Parent Program is organized into three divisions: day treatment, outpatient, and consultation and education. Paraprofessional staff members are involved in a number of different clinical functions within each of these three divisions.

The day treatment and outpatient staff members use therapeutic methods based on the principles of behavior therapy to treat families, children, and adolescents with behavior disorders. The staff members who provide the clinical services also are responsible for the consultation and education activities. As a consequence, these staff members are able to teach their personal clinical skills both to agencies requesting consultation and education services and to the general public.

This teaching occurs in a series of prevention-oriented mental health education courses. With the exception of most of the consultation and education services to agencies, all the activities of the Child and Parent Program take place at the center headquarters.

Background

Madison County is the wealthiest in Alabama; 50% of the families have annual incomes of $14,000 or more. A large National Aeronautic and Space Administration research center is located in Huntsville, and, consequently, many highly educated people live in the area. About 23% of the catchment district residents live in rural areas. About 15% of catchment district residents are black; most remaining residents are white.

*Contact: Huntsville-Madison County Mental Health Center
          660 Gallatin Street, S. W.
          Huntsville, Alabama   35801
          205/533-1970
          Attention: Roger Rinn, Director, Children's Services

In 1970, the center was small and traditional. In 1971, Jack Turner (Ph.D.) and William H. Goodson (M.D.) received a three-year grant from the National Institute of Mental Health to create the first community mental health center based on the system-wide application of behavior modification practices (except for cases requiring chemotherapy). The center grew rapidly in size, success, and national recognition, and currently seven other community mental health centers in this country are applying the Huntsville model. The approach may also be adopted by some mental health facilities in Mexico.

The center places an unusually heavy emphasis on research. In the past year (1976), 16 professional papers and four books were written by center staff members. The research material is written up after working hours, usually by the professional staff members, but the paraprofessional staff members are encouraged to participate and are listed as co-authors on investigations to which they contribute.

The center operates from one large headquarters on an annual budget of $1,310,000 (fiscal year ending September 30, 1976). About 43% of the budget comes from federal sources, about 35% from local funds, and about 22% from state sources. The center employs 19 professionals and 17 paraprofessionals in service (nonadministrative) roles. The center also employs three nurses.

Philosophically, the entire Huntsville Center[1] is oriented towards using therapeutic and administrative methods based on the behavioral approach. Behavior therapy involves a service delivery approach that emphasizes the use of evidence that can be objectively observed, measured, and reported. This is in contrast to many other therapeutic strategies that tend to measure change or progress by relying solely on the subjective judgment of the people involved. An example of the behavior therapy approach is a contract by a parent to ignore the whining behavior demonstrated by his/her children. The relevant evidence in this case, is the rate (increase, decrease) of whining behavior displayed by the children.

The behavioral approach was chosen for use at Huntsville not only because the staff believes it works, but because the staff values the clear and accurate reporting of results in accountability reports. It is a method that emphasizes competence in its employees (performance can be measured through observation and record keeping) rather than academic degrees. Thus, at Huntsville, behavior modification is viewed as an effective, efficient approach to community mental health that costs less and yields more.

The behavior modification approach involves a practical set of procedures that is appealing and accessible to paraprofessionals as well as to many profes-

[1]For a fuller description of the Huntsville Center, see Turner, A. J., Goodson, W. H., and Rinn, R. C. *The Huntsville model: Accountability in community mental health.* Cambridge, Massachusetts: Research Media, in press.

sionals. The high degree of planning and structure involved in using behavior modification techniques may be helpful in preventing paraprofessionals from making mistakes, and in providing these staff members with a realistic, encouraging sense of progress.

The program staff members teach families to set their own goals and to reward themselves for the achievement of these goals. In addition, the day treatment staff members set academic and behavioral goals for each child, with little concrete input from the families. The practices employed with clients are also used with the center staff members. Center employees (including all paraprofessionals) set work goals and receive recognition and salary raises for high achievement. In fact, the center applies the behavioral approach to all levels of its operation and to all of its clinical services.

Originally, the Huntsville Center provided direct services to adults, with minimal service for children. The center wanted to offer more comprehensive services to its clients, and in May 1975, Dr. Roger Rinn, the current Child and Parent Director and a center staff member since 1971, developed the Child and Parent Program in accordance with behavior modification practices.

The Child and Parent Program occupies a part of one wing in the three-wing Huntsville Center. It is a small space which contributes to a family feeling, enhancing the group solidarity of the program. The day treatment paraprofessional staff members do not have offices; as "teachers," they are accustomed to carrying out their work at desks in classrooms, after the children leave or before the children arrive. All offices (with the exception of the day treatment classrooms) open into a spacious corridor that serves as a waiting room for clients and as a gathering space for Child and Parent staff during infrequent breaks.

The Child and Parent Program spends $411,000 annually, or about 30% of the total center budget. The program employs seven professionals and seven paraprofessionals in service roles. Most of the paraprofessionals in the center have baccalaureate degrees. Salaries for professionals range from $10,500 to $25,000 annually. Salaries for paraprofessionals range from $7,500 to $11,000 annually. Annual expenditures for Child and Parent professionals in service functions are about $85,000. For paraprofessionals, this figure is about $67,000.

The program each year serves 62 clients in its day treatment division, 699 clients in its outpatient division, and 15 agencies through its consultation and education division. The consultation and education division, furthermore, serves around 90 participants annually in 14 mental health education courses.

Because it does not receive federal research or training grants, the Child and Parent Program must meet expenses with the funds normally available to any community mental health center. The mental health education courses offered, for a fee, by program professionals to the public are self-supporting. The day treatment program receives service funds from sources established by federal Title XX legislation and from client fees. The family therapy outpatient clinic receives fees from noninsured fee-paying clients and reimbursements from insurance or state sources for insured or needy clients. Community consultation activities bring clients to the program but are probably not self-supporting.

Program Organization and Services

Recordkeeping procedures are essential to the operation of all divisions of the Child and Parent program. As an example, the day treatment coordinator (a professional) receives points and rewards for the performance of the day treatment unit. Accordingly, the coordinator is motivated to promote optimal performance from the paraprofessionals in the unit. Because they receive points and rewards for competent performance, the paraprofessionals are also motivated to achieve high standards.

The day treatment division (and thus its director) is responsible for achieving the outcome (end product) and the process (intermediate steps) goals that have been established for the division. The outcome goals involve teaching the children various new behaviors and replacing less desirable behaviors with new habits and skills. One process goal is to develop and implement procedures for assessing the progress of the children in meeting behavioral and academic goals. Another process goal is to send frequent reports to the professional who referred the given child for day treatment. The day treatment paraprofessionals receive time off each day to maintain their records and to show them to the day treatment coordinator during the supervisory sessions.

The program's services form a partially interlocking structure. The outpatient division provides therapy services to families, parents, and children or adolescents. Parents of children enrolled in the day treatment program may be referred in turn to the outpatient division for services, although most receive treatment from the coordinator of the day treatment division. The consultation and education division makes referrals from community agencies to the day treatment and outpatient divisions. In addition, day treatment and outpatient professionals (and one paraprofessional) teach behavior modification skills to persons employed by various agencies.

Several unusual features contribute to the success of the program. A record keeping service, staffed entirely by paraprofessionals, processes and scores the numerous forms used to evaluate staff performance. The secretaries in the waiting-room area are trained to create an accepting, friendly atmosphere for clients and to make relevant observations (e.g., of a parent hitting a child) for outpatient therapists. The senior program professionals, Drs.

Roger Rinn and Allan Markle, have developed parent education and achievement motivation training courses.[2]

Consultation and Education Division.   Consultation and education services are organized into a three-phase approach involving case consultation, on-the-job training, and consultation by program staff for difficulties arising after agency personnel have completed the training.[3] As the result of consultation and education efforts, the seven probation officers in the county court system have, over the past four years, taught more than 1,400 parents the skills contained in the parent education course developed by Dr. Rinn.

While most agency consultation and education services are provided by professionals, this division does maintain a paraprofessional staff member who is a baccalaureate certified teacher in the county school system. The school system pays 80% of her salary. She helps teachers with classroom management techniques and also makes referrals to the program's day treatment and outpatient division. Maintaining a consultant within a school system is feasible only where a large volume of problems requiring consultation exists.

Professional staff members from the program offer seven different prevention-oriented mental health education programs to the general public (e.g., positive parenting training, assertiveness training). Labeled as "courses," these programs provide nonstigmatizing opportunities for promotion of mental health and attract enrollees who might not seek therapy.

Outpatient Division.   A paraprofessional performs interviewing and testing "intake" functions for the outpatient division. Additionally, until he earned his master's degree, a paraprofessional with a bachelor's degree in psychology acted successfully as an outpatient therapist. He has since been

[2]The principles taught in the parent education courses are presented in Rinn, R. C. & Markle, A. *Positive parenting.* Cambridge, Massachusetts: Research Media, Inc., 1977. Research demonstrating its efficacy is found in Rinn, R. C., Vernon, J. C., & Wise, M. J. Training parents of behaviorally disordered children in groups: A three years' program evaluation. *Behavior Therapy,* 1975, *6,* 378–387. The course for underachieving students is fully described in Markle, A., Rinn, R. C., & Worthy, M. *Achievement motivation training: Helping the underachieving student* (book submitted for publication, 1977). The efficacy of the achievement motivation program has been documented in Markle, A. & Rinn, R. C. Achievement motivation training in a community mental health center: A preliminary report (manuscript submitted for publication, 1977).

[3]This model is described in Rinn, R. C. Consultation and education services for agencies: Process and evaluation, a chapter in Turner, A. J., Goodson, W. H., & Rinn, R. C. *The Huntsville model: Accountability in community mental health* (Cambridge, Massachusetts: Research Media, in press).

promoted to professional status. Currently, one paraprofessional (aside from the intake worker) is an outpatient therapist.

Day Treatment Division.   The ultimate goal of the day treatment division is to teach children, ages 5–15, the academic and behavioral skills necessary for a successful return to the school situation. Decisions on whether to place the children in the day treatment setting are made by a screening committee comprised of the program's B.A.-level consultant, the paraprofessional staff members in the day treatment program, and the day treatment coordinator (chairperson).

Children are placed by age and academic achievement scores into one of three small classes, averaging eight students in size. In two of the classes, two paraprofessionals are responsible for the children. One paraprofessional, called a "teacher," is responsible for the academic skills of each child. The teacher places special emphasis on reading and communication skills. The other paraprofessional, called a "counselor," is responsible for the classroom behaviors, such as being in one's seat or working on tasks. In conferences with the day treatment coordinator, the paraprofessionals set specific, measurable goals for the children. The teachers and counselors emphasize rewards for desirable behavior, and especially use tokens that the children can exchange for a variety of treats such as candy or recess.

Use of Paraprofessionals

Since paraprofessionals can often do as competent a job for less money than professional staff members, the Huntsville Center hires paraprofessionals as outpatient therapists, day treatment counselors or teachers, or school-based consultants. Thus, the center can deliver essential services while still remaining within its budget. Another reason for using paraprofessionals is that they are considered to be more willing and eager to perform the repetitive and difficult clinical tasks that may cause a professional to look for a job elsewhere. Finally, the Huntsville people feel that paraprofessionals are more likely to "know what they don't know and to be willing to learn." The fact that the behavior modification approach *emphasizes competencies rather than credentials* makes the Huntsville Center a congenial working environment for paraprofessionals.

Consultation and Education.   The paraprofessional in this division is on the staff of the county schools. This teacher-consultant is knowledgeable about the school system as well as about the behavior modification techniques used by the program. The school personnel identify her as being a part of the school rather than as an "outsider" from the community mental health center; as a consequence, she is more readily approached by teachers experiencing difficulties and is more able to collaborate with teachers in developing treatment programs in the regular classrooms.

Her job involves rotating among schools as a mental health specialist and working within classrooms to help teachers who encounter difficulties with individual children. In addition to helping the teachers directly, she also attempts to teach her mental health skills to teachers. This paraprofessional staff member also acts as a liaison between the school and the day treatment division of the program; in this role she makes referrals, introduces the children to the day treatment activities, and reintroduces discharged children to the school setting.

Outpatient.   The Associate of Arts-level intake worker in this division divides her time equally between intake interviews and formal testing. She administers these tests: WISC-R, Bender, WAIS, Achievement Motivation Imagery, and the Family Interest Test. This worker gathers information useful to the professional (M. A.- and Ph.D.-level) therapists and in some cases may make decisions on whether to refer the client to a professional therapist in the center. Generally, however, she consults her supervisor on referral decisions. This paraprofessional also assists in training teachers to teach the Achievement Motivation Training Course developed through the program. She has also performed pre- and post-testing in a research study on the effects of the Achievement Motivation course. Another paraprofessional (bachelor's level) acts as a therapist in the outpatient division. She employs all the skills required of professional staff in conducting behavioral family therapy. Moreover, she performs comprehensive intake interviews, sets goals for families, and develops treatment programs for ameliorating maladaptive behavior.

Day Treatment.   Paraprofessionals devote about one-third of each day to administrative duties such as formulating treatment plans, charting the progress of the children, maintaining contacts with the teachers and parents of the children, and meeting with the day treatment coordinator in daily hour-long group supervisory sessions to discuss strategies for individual children. The remaining time, about five hours daily, is spent with the children.

The children in the day treatment program are "difficult" and require patience, energy, and those working with them need the ability to relate to children in a playful yet firm fashion. The paraprofessional staff members often feel they are particularly well qualified for this task, as they were selected on the basis of relevant skills rather than degrees. The paraprofessional staff members in this division often feel that the academic classroom training of professionals does not necessarily prepare them for these tasks. While the paraprofessional staff members find their work to be stimulating and meaningful, some of them remarked that many professional staff members might find day treatment teaching and counseling duties to be boring and repetitive. While interacting with the children, the paraprofessionals simultaneously and consistently implement a detailed treatment plan. At the end of their challenging and demanding days, these staff members are usually quite tired.

The paraprofessional staff members will pay home visits when such visits are deemed necessary (once in every seven or eight cases) to achieve the treatment plans. In such cases, the parents can become more active partners in treatment. In addition, the paraprofessionals routinely contact parents at the beginning and termination of treatment, to facilitate cooperation and communication between the program and the home.

To date, the day treatment coordinator has been a professional. However, the coordinator believes that this role could be handled by an experienced, intelligent, and clinically skilled paraprofessional.

Recruitment

The center seeks paraprofessionals who are eager to learn and who can understand abstractions. Paraprofessionals are encouraged to read research reports and (through flexible work hours, when feasible) to work toward higher academic degrees. Most new paraprofessionals do have B.A. or B.S. degrees, although not necessarily in the behavioral sciences. The center administration believes that a college degree indicates that the individual is able to discipline himself in a learning situation. Although the job market is flooded with personnel possessing master's degrees, the center will not hire them to fill paraprofessional slots. The center recognizes that any new employee (with the exception of those with fieldwork experience in behavior modification) will require special training at the center; furthermore, the center staff members believe that master's-level people are more likely to vacate paraprofessional-level jobs. (The center's policy, instead, is to attempt to provide professional-level staff positions for qualified staff paraprofessionals who have earned master's degrees.)

The Child and Parent Program's seven service-oriented paraprofessionals currently are all women, averaging age 26. One paraprofessional is black; the others are white. Most of the paraprofessionals are natives of Huntsville or Madison County.

Selection

The first program coordinators, all professionals, were selected by Dr. Roger Rinn, the program director. Dr. Rinn very deliberately picked competent coordinators whose interests and outlooks were similar to his own. In short, he hired people whom he liked and with whom he could work effectively. In consultation with Dr. Rinn, these coordinators in turn selected the paraprofessionals in their divisions. Presently all prospective paraprofessional employees are interviewed by the program administrator, who is familiar with all the job duties in the program. People meeting the program's standards (described in the next paragraph) are then interviewed by the coordinator of the division in which the opening exists. The administrator and the coordinator jointly pick a finalist, who is interviewed very briefly by the program director. The director almost always approves the candidates submitted to him.

The selection standards for professionals and paraprofessionals are identical, except that plans to seek a higher educational degree increase a paraprofessional's (and even an M.A.-level professional's) chances of being hired. The interviewers do not look for passive, conforming paraprofessionals; rather they seek paraprofessionals who, like the program professionals, are assertive, eager to learn, and enjoy working with children and teenagers. It is also quite important that candidates be likable, socially skilled, cheerful, and able to be direct in expressing feelings. All candidates are judged on their attitudes toward accountable working conditions and toward behavior modification. They must value the maintenance of detailed records and believe that mental health services require ongoing evaluation and improvement. They must also be willing to be judged and rewarded by merit pay increases and social recognition on the basis of their performance.

Training

All new employees (regardless of degree level or job duties) receive the same orientation training together. The training is provided by the center for all programs and is given over an eight-week period of time, for two to three hours daily. Thus, employees work part-time while they receive training. Employees, however, do not negotiate job duties with their supervisors until they complete orientation training, for the training helps to provide them with the skills and knowledge required for negotiation.

The center's orientation program is comprehensive and involves a number of approaches to teaching and learning. The orientation program includes a competency training course that demonstrates behavior modification principles through concrete experiences, such as making a contract to stop smoking. It also includes an assertiveness training course that prepares new staff members to negotiate task description contracts with their supervisors.

The Child and Parent Program supplements the orientation training provided by the center with specialized training that relates to the program. For example, the paraprofessional intake worker is trained by her supervisor to administer tests to children. New employees receive intensive supervision and are also encouraged by their supervisors to ask questions.

For in-service training, paraprofessionals may voluntarily attend any of the 45 seminars offered annually by the center. The seminars are offered free of charge and are open to both the professional and paraprofessional staff members. Paraprofessionals do not receive academic credit for orientation or in-service training experiences.

Supervision

The objective ratings on the Huntsville evaluation forms (see "Evaluation" later in this chapter) are supplemented by scheduled or informal conversations between employees and their supervisors. These conversations enable the supervisor and the paraprofessional or professional supervisee to discuss the ratings on the comprehensive forms and to focus on issues related to client progress. As employees gain in experience and are less likely to commit mistakes, the scheduled supervision is provided less frequently and focuses primarily on difficult cases rather than on routine matters.

Mobility

The program and the center actively encourage paraprofessionals to upgrade their skills through formal education. Employees are allowed to take time off from work to attend classes, but usually are required to make up this time. The center will promote to professional-level slots qualified staff paraprofessionals who have earned master's degrees while working at the center. Applications for relevant openings are first taken in-house, and the position is given to the most highly qualified professional or paraprofessional applicant. Because professional-level slots infrequently become available within the center, the vertical mobility of paraprofessionals at Huntsville is limited.

One program paraprofessional was helped by several center professionals on his master's thesis. Abiding by the requirements that apply to program professionals, he first submitted his proposal to the center's research committee. Judging that his proposal adhered to ethical guidelines and was relevant to the goals of the center, the committee gave him permission to use the center's records in his research. One senior program professional helped the paraprofessional with statistical problems, and another senior center professional provided assistance with conceptual issues. Thus, highly experienced professionals from the center served essentially as thesis advisors to this paraprofessional staff member.

Because of the very low turnover rate, the program rarely is faced with the need to hire paraprofessionals to fill existing slots. New jobs result when new positions are created, and then center personnel are alerted prior to "going public." Unless an outside applicant is more qualified by virtue of training and experience, the position will be given to the most qualified center employee who applies within the seven-day deadline for in-house transfers. This practice boosts the morale of center paraprofessionals, who can look forward to future job changes as paraprofessionals, as well as to possible upward mobility. Slots not filled by the center staff are usually filled by the most capable persons who have served internships or practicums at the center while pursuing bachelor's degrees. The practice of hiring interns enables the program to employ paraprofessionals with previous experience in behavioral therapy. Furthermore, this practice enables the center (or program) staff members to know who they are hiring and to employ paraprofessionals who enjoy the behavioral approach and know what to expect from the work. The program does not actively recruit paraprofessionals in the community.

Status and Morale

Despite unhappiness over what are felt to be inadequate salaries, morale is very high among the paraprofessional staff members at Huntsville. What accounts for the high level of morale?

The basic cause seems to be that the paraprofessional personnel can and do express positive and negative feelings directly to all professionals, including the program director. Complaints are usually specific and, thus, can be handled in a constructive fashion. Furthermore, paraprofessionals feel very free to ask professionals for advice about work-related and personal problems.

Other elements that contribute to the high morale are a positive atmosphere in the program; professional staff members who don't "pull rank"; and the easy interaction between the professional and paraprofessional staff members—the sense that they are "all on the same team."

Almost all staff members, professional and paraprofessional, show considerable pride in their individual work and in the efforts of the Child and Parent Program. Competency, not degree level, is the ultimate criterion for self-respect and public recognition. The program is seen as being "fair" to the employees—each person is rewarded through merit pay hikes and social recognition and recognized for conscientious, competent work. Paraprofessionals are valued by the center as competent service providers who can deliver needed services at reduced costs. Center and program professionals expressed almost total satisfaction with the performance of paraprofessionals. Clients rarely raise difficulties concerning the paraprofessionals' degree status. The only complaint of staff professionals was that paraprofessionals are less interested in research and in keeping up with the literature.

Pressures external to the catchment district, however, are causing the center to reduce the number of paraprofessionals employed and, thus, to reduce the quantity of services available to the public. The center professionals maintain that restrictions on third-party payments (especially by the federal Title XX program) comprise the most potent external pressure. Additional restricting factors are sections of PL 94–63 (the 1975 federal Community Mental Health legislation) dealing with qualifications for outpatient therapists, and sections of Alabama state legal codes.

The use of paraprofessionals is also restricted by factors unique to the Huntsville catchment district. These factors do not necessarily apply to other localities. Huntsville is a community where an unusually high percentage of residents possess baccalaureate or graduate degrees. Some center professionals believe that some Huntsville residents prefer to receive services from people who are their peers or superiors in terms of educational level. As a result of perceived local conditions, the program often places professionals in positions requiring a high level of visibility or responsibility (e.g., program director).

An example of an exception to this low-profile rule involves an outpatient therapist who worked with program clients and their families one-to-one for two years prior to receiving his M.A. in psychology. This therapist only rarely experienced difficulties related to his degree status. He discovered that clients respect competency and genuine interest rather than external degrees. As an ethical person, he introduced himself as "Mr." and always answered truthfully if questioned about his degree level. Most clients continued to accept his services after discovering that he was a paraprofessional. On rare occasions when clients voiced concern about his degree, he always referred them to a program professional.

Evaluation

The Huntsville approach to evaluation is unusually thorough. The general features, if not the specific details of this approach, are applicable to centers that do not adhere to the principles of behavior modification.

At many community mental health centers, the staff members are evaluated every six to 12 months by a supervisor who simply completes a check list. Service delivery programs may not be evaluated at all. Such periodic and impressionistic evaluation may or may not be accurate. Even if accurate, this approach to evaluation enables programs and employees systematically to correct mistakes and to improve performance only at widely spaced intervals.

At the Huntsville Center, however, evaluation is carried out on an ongoing daily or weekly basis jointly by the staff members along with their supervisor. Furthermore, the evaluation is objective (descriptive of measurable behavior both of clients and of staff members) rather than intuitive in nature. The evaluation data, thus, serve as information indicative of areas of strength, and of areas in which individual or program performance can be improved.

Outcome evaluation measures compare observed or reported changes from the baserate of problem behavior with the changes required to achieve the goal set by or for the client.[4] The center has not systematically compared the performance of professional and paraprofessional clinicians in achieving outcome goals.

Day treatment outcome evaluation data directly reflect the performance of paraprofessionals, for paraprofessionals perform almost all direct clinical services in this division. Paraprofessionals routinely observe and chart the

[4]The statistical measure of percentage of goal attainment is:

$$\frac{(\text{Median outcome frequency}) - (\text{Median baserate frequency})}{(\text{Goal}) - (\text{Median baserate frequency})} \times 100$$

behavior of the children. The day treatment coordinator, if he wishes, can check the accuracy of these ratings through observations of his own. Averaging across the three highest priority goals, day treatment counselors achieve a 93% success rate. Using the same measurement, day treatment teachers achieve an 84% success rate.

Such data have not been gathered on the paraprofessional intake worker in the outpatient division. The school-based paraprofessional is 84% effective in achieving the stated goals.[5]

Supervisees (whether paraprofessional or professional) negotiate with their supervisors the point value of routine recordkeeping and follow-up tasks. The points received for these routine items are summed as one line items on a more comprehensive form detailing the duties that accompany a job. Generally, supervisees do not have much leeway over determining specific job duties, but do exert an influence on the number of points received for successful completion of these duties.

The points received on the comprehensive forms are reviewed annually by supervisors as the basis for administering competency-based rewards to both paraprofessionals and professionals. When funds are available (as in four of the past five years) performance-related monetary rewards are allocated.

This system is carefully designed to promote competent performance, while avoiding possible harm to clients or unfair outcomes to supervisees. Supervisees are kept aware of their performance frequently during the year and compete against their own baserate performance. Client progress is not included as a job description item. At Huntsville it is felt that the inclusion of client progress items might encourage clinicians to set client goals that could too readily be accomplished.

In Conclusion

The Child and Parent Program at the Huntsville-Madison County Mental Health Center uses principles of behavior modification in all aspects of its operation: administration, staff, evaluation, and service delivery. Accordingly, the program is able to emphasize accountability, by recording the activities and measuring the performance of staff members, and able to promote empiricism, by charting the progress achieved by clients. Paraprofessionals participate in all three of the program's divisions: day care, outpatient, and consultation and education. The associated staff training, supervision, and evaluation procedures are specific and concrete; the paraprofessionals at Huntsville find this

[5]This effectiveness figure represents an average of two statistics: (1) the percentage approximation to the goal of reducing problems of one-third of clients to preset levels; (2) the percentage of clients referred to the mental health center receiving services within 30 days of referral.

emphasis on results to be congenial and nonmystifying. Staff members are rewarded for current competent performance rather than for degrees earned previously; the paraprofessionals at Huntsville respect this orientation and find it to be equitable. Paraprofessionals receive extensive training and supervision. Given the availability of relevant positions, this education allows them to assume additional responsibilities following the mastery of the appropriate skills. The data gathered by the Child and Parent Program indicate that paraprofessionals are highly effective in performing their functions.

Chapter 5

CONSULTATION AND EDUCATION SERVICES

INTRODUCTION

Description of the Service Area

Consultation and Education was one of the five services required by the original community mental health centers legislation. Programs in this area are unique in that direct services to individual clients are not involved. Because of the pressing needs for direct clinical services, many mental health centers had neglected the development of their consultation and education programs. Consequently, the 1975 Community Mental Health Center Amendments include special supplemental consultation and education funding.

One goal of consultation and education programs is to provide indirect services to catchment area residents by assisting community providers of mental health and related services to enhance their competency. Providers include, but are not limited to, health professionals, schools, courts, law enforcement and correctional agencies, members of the clergy, public welfare agencies, and physical health delivery agencies. Consultation services characteristically are offered when providers experience problems with individual clients, program development efforts, or administrative concerns. Education services for providers, in contrast, are less frequently problem-centered, may be structured as a course, and can function as an in-service training experience.

While consultation services are offered primarily to providers, education services are generally offered both to providers and to the wider community.

The more specific functions for which a consultation and education program is responsible include fostering coordination of mental health services among various entities in the catchment area; promoting the prevention and control of rape and proper treatment of victims of rape; increasing the visibility, identifiability, and accessibility of the community mental health center; and distributing and disseminating mental health information for the purposes of increasing awareness about mental health problems, promoting positive mental health, and reducing the frequency of mental health problems.

Selection of the Site Visited

The recommendations for consultation and education programs were obtained from regional Department of Health, Education, and Welfare offices, as well as from several mental health professionals familiar with this service area.

In-depth telephone interviews were conducted with the directors of ten consultation and education programs that made extensive use of paraprofessionals. Most of these ten programs are separate service units; however, in many mental health centers these indirect services are delivered by staff members of direct service units.

Some of the consultation and education programs surveyed operated in relative autonomy from the remaining programs in the community health center. Other consultation and education programs collaborated to some extent with various center programs in providing referrals, sharing staff, or implementing publicity and outreach activities.

Consultation services are offered to a wide array of catchment area service providers. However, services are usually requested or offered to professional persons (such as psychologists or schoolteachers), while nonprofessional persons (such as administrators of grass roots community organizations) are not typically recipients.

Education services both to providers and to the community tend to be short-term and informal rather than long-term and systematic. While the programs surveyed engage in efforts to educate the community about the mental health center, most of the programs do not use their community contacts to provide information about the community to the mental health center. Although the programs devote some effort to coordination of mental health services among community entities, this goal is not typically a high priority item. Rape prevention and treatment efforts are offered only by some of the programs surveyed.

Even though most of the centers surveyed are providing the minimal services required by law and receive special supplementary funding, consultation and education does not appear to be a highly developed service area. Our survey suggests that community mental health centers generally do not offer a systematically planned and integrated array of consultation and education services designed both to treat and to prevent the development of mental health problems within the catchment district.

The number of paraprofessionals in consultation and education programs is usually small, generally not exceeding four. The paraprofessionals perform a wide variety of services, specializing particularly in providing education and other services to community citizens in community settings. Most programs surveyed had not developed procedures for training professionals or paraprofessionals in the complex set of skills involved in mental health consultation. Some programs give consultation assignments to paraprofessionals and professionals without distinction, while other programs allow only professionals, or perhaps professionals and bachelor level paraprofessionals, to provide consultation services. A contributing factor to reliance on professionals is the belief that recipients prefer not to receive consultative assistance from persons with less formal education than they have.

The Dr. Solomon Carter Fuller Community Mental Health Center in Boston, Massachusetts, was selected as the site of our case study in the consultation and education service area. This consultation and education program offers a wide array of services to many types of providers, both from public agencies and from grass roots organizations. Many of these services are designed for special age or ethnic groups. Paraprofessionals participate fully in the delivery of most services, often working on an equal-status basis in teams with professionals. Furthermore, the paraprofessionals are carefully selected and trained by the program. The program differs from most of those surveyed in that: (1) its director is a paraprofessional from the local community; (2) paraprofessionals routinely and frequently provide consultation and education services to a wide variety of professionals; (3) paraprofessionals as community representatives design some of the services offered by the program; (4) in addition to educating the community about the center, the program systematically educates the mental health center about the community; and (5) the original staff members were selected jointly by community residents and by professionals. The viability of the approach is documented by the fact that the program has continued in an effective manner since its inception in 1970.

DR. SOLOMON CARTER FULLER COMMUNITY MENTAL HEALTH CENTER: A CASE STUDY IN CONSULTATION AND EDUCATION SERVICES*

The Dr. Solomon Carter Fuller Community Mental Health Center is part of the Massachusetts Department of Mental Health and is affiliated with the

*Contact: Dr. Solomon Carter Fuller Community Mental Health Center
85 East Newton Street
Boston, Massachusetts 02118
617/266-8800
Attention: Frieda Garcia, Director, Consultation & Education Program

Boston University Medical School. It serves a catchment district of 116,000 citizens (1970 census) in Boston, Massachusetts. There are four distinct neighborhoods in the district—Roxbury, North Dorchester, South End, and the Back Bay—and they differ considerably in terms of the ethnic background, age, living situation, and income characteristics of their residents. The population of the catchment district has a high proportion of ethnic minorities—48% black; 41% white; 7% Spanish-speaking (Hispanic); and 4% "other minorities." These percentages represent the 1970 census. The black and Hispanic populations are the fastest growing segment of the population and are underrepresented by these figures. Other minority groups are also seriously underrepresented by the census statistics. The population is faced with many urban stresses, such as poverty, blighted housing, and high unemployment, which contribute to a high need for and use of mental health services.

The Consultation and Education (C & E) program is one of many programs at the Fuller Center. Of the center's service staff hours, about 49% involve mental health professionals; 15% involve activities by nurses; 17% are performed by people with B.A. degrees; and 19% are executed by sub-B.A. staff. At present the C & E program employs 43 staff members: 23 are service delivery paraprofessionals, 9.5 are service delivery professionals, and the remainder are clerical employees. About 16 of the paraprofessionals reside within the catchment district. This is in contrast to the program's professional staff members, most of whom reside outside the district.

Unlike most of the center's programs, the C & E program is entirely supported by a federal staffing grant, administered by the state of Massachusetts through the center. (Recently, the federal grant came to an end; however, the state is continuing funding at its previous level.) This special grant allows the center to make an unusually strong commitment to C & E work. Approximately 7% (February 1975) of the total center's staff hours are devoted to C & E activities. In March 1975, the C & E unit provided about 60% of the total center consultation staff hours; the remaining consultation activities were carried out by other programs. All programs (including C & E) within the mental health center are under the jurisdiction of an "area board," a community group comprised of residents from the catchment district, and of a board of trustees, whose membership is partially determined by the area board.

A consultation and education program traditionally provides *indirect* services to the public agencies and grass roots organizations in a catchment district, thus helping the staff members of these local groups to provide more effective direct services to their clients, the community residents. Traditional C & E services, furthermore, include increasing the awareness of community members and organizations as to the kind of services provided by the mental health center, assistance in early case identification, and implementation of primary prevention work. This chapter describes how C & E paraprofessionals at the Fuller Center design and deliver the traditional consultation and education services, both autonomously and cooperatively with professionals. The chapter also considers how the paraprofessionals and professionals design and deliver additional direct services needed by the community, and how a C & E program can bridge a wide gap between a politically aware community (with a history of involvement in War on Poverty programs) and a professional center. Numerous examples of the resulting programs will be described.

The C & E program staff members describe their program as being the most "community oriented" one in the center. The staff members educate the community about the center, a traditional C & E function, but also perform the unusual function of educating the other center staff members about the community. The program offers direct and indirect services at community locations to local agencies, grass roots organizations, and loosely knit groupings of community clients. Professionals and paraprofessionals work side by side on the same tasks; the program's director, in fact, has a bachelor's degree and resides within the catchment district.

Most program professionals, representing a variety of disciplines, and all paraprofessional service personnel are assigned to one of two teams and spend about 50% of their time at team headquarters located in the community rather than in the central facility. The director spends about 50% of her time in community settings, serving on various boards whose activities relate to community issues. The team members deliver services in the team headquarters, as well as in community settings. As team members, paraprofessionals consult with agencies and also provide services directly to community clients.

The more experienced service personnel spend about 25% of their time in the center building, collaborating with staff members from other center programs on service delivery efforts. In these collaborative efforts, C & E staff members provide technical assistance and thus enable other center programs to provide services that are more community-oriented in nature.

C & E staff members spend their remaining time with internal units responsible for the administrative-coordination system of the C & E program. As unit members, paraprofessionals are involved in planning activities to be carried out by their specific unit. The units also plan and implement services that assist the C & E program itself and the Fuller Center. Both the units and the teams have been part of the program since its inception, although both structures have undergone changes during the history of the program.

Background

The Fuller Community Mental Health Center was established in 1969 with a federal staffing grant. The grant was secured by Dr. Bernard Bandler of the Boston University Medical School along with Dr. William Malumud and others. Dr. Bandler's grant proposal deliberately requested funds to establish a full C & E program before asking for funds for the additional staff members needed to supplement the existing programs in the other four traditional service areas (outpatient, inpatient, day treatment, and emergency). Dr. Bandler's concept of community mental health prompted him to use the C & E. program as an initial vehicle for developing trust and communication between the center and the community.[1]

All original C & E staff members, including the director, were hired following their approval by two independent committees. One committee consisted of community residents, the other of medical school professionals. Each committee had veto power over the choices of the other committee. The original director, Ms. Ruth Batson, was a community activist who resided (and continues to reside) within the center's catchment district. This fact increased the program's credibility within the community. In addition, Ms. Batson, a paraprofessional, was appointed to a tenured associate professorship in Boston University's Department of Psychiatry, indicating the extent to which the knowledge and experience of community members is of value to mental health professionals.

Ms. Batson directed the C & E program until 1975. Having successfully completed the difficult task of creating a viable and innovative program, she left to focus on a new challenge. She secured a grant to explore the involvement of mental health institutions in crisis situations (such as the then-current desegregation of the Boston schools) and became director of Boston University's Crisis Intervention Program. She has since earned a master's degree.

In February, 1975, Ms. Frieda Garcia became the new director of the C & E program. A member of the catchment district's most rapidly growing minority population (Hispanic), Ms. Garcia is a Dominican-American. She resides within the catchment district. Ms. Garcia was hired through a search process that involved the Massachusetts Department of Mental Health, the center's area board, the Boston University New Careers Program, and the C & E staff members. Currently, the C & E program is attempting to secure for Ms. Garcia, who has a B.A. degree, an associate professorship appointment at Boston University. It should be considered that the similarities in the selection processes and qualifications of Ms. Garcia and Ms. Batson may account, in part, for the smooth leadership transition within the C & E program and for the continuing viability of the C & E program within the center.

Strong and friendly ties between the community and the program were established during Ms. Batson's tenure and have been retained under Ms. Garcia's leadership. Both directors also have contributed to the strong sense of pride and solidarity felt by C & E program staff members.

Launched as part of a Boston University program that later became the Fuller Center, the C & E program helped to focus a community demand for services not yet available from the center. Although funding constraints delayed the establishment of new programs, the C & E program had contributed

---

[1]The history and philosophy of the C & E program are described in detail in the chapter by Bandler, Batson, and Peters, in *Paraprofessionals in mental health: Theory and practice,* the companion volume to this book

to increased consciousness within the community. As other programs became established in the center, the C & E program continued to see itself as the community advocate within the center—a position described by a staff member as "in but not of the center."

Community-oriented suggestions for changes in treatment and training were not always welcomed by existing understaffed services. Therefore, the C & E program's relationship to other center programs has been lukewarm or combative at times during its history.

About a year after Ms. Garcia was hired as director, the new C & E program moved its administrative offices into a building which contained most center programs. To some extent, the struggles of the early years have resulted in community advocacy being viewed as a resource for the rest of the center, and a new collaborative spirit between the C & E program and the other center programs is now emerging.

Overall, the C & E program has been helping other service programs to become aware of existing community resources and needs. For example, C & E staff members are helping the inpatient program personnel to identify community resources that make it possible to transfer patients from the inpatient wards of the center to appropriate community locations. Occasionally, other programs within the center will take over activities initiated by the C & E staff. An example of such an activity is a community apartment established by the C & E program for three discharged mental patients; this shared apartment arrangement enables staff members from the mental health center to provide services to all three clients during a single visit.

Currently the C & E program employs the following staff members in service functions: two psychiatrists (plus a half-time position); four Ph.D. psychologists; three M.S.W.s; one R.N.; four B.A.-level service personnel; and about 19 sub-B.A.-level service personnel.

The annual salary range for professionals is: M.D.s: $28,883–$32,262; Ph.D.s (Psychology): $15,410–$19,591; M.S.W. clinical supervisor: $13,813–$17,573; M.S.W.s: $11,570–$14,658; mental health nurses: $12,373–$15,602. Three B.A.-level job slots exist; B.A. salary levels range from $9,622 to $14,658 annually. Only two sub-B.A. career levels exist, severely limiting the vertical mobility of sub-B.A. employees. The sub-B.A. salaries range from $7,199 to $11,775 annually. Currently only two sub-B.A. employees are classified at the higher career level.

The budget for the Fuller Center during fiscal year 1976–77 was $5.5 million. The budget for the C & E program during this period was about $523,000; about $215,000 was spent for the salaries of full-time professional service staff members, while about $225,000 was provided for the salaries of full-time C & E paraprofessional service staff members. In June 1977, the federal staffing grant to the C & E program expired; at that time the funding for the program was continued at the previous level by the state of Massachusetts.

Program Organization and Services

The C & E program is organized into five units, each of which is responsible for activities in specific areas. Three of these units are responsible for activities carried out primarily in community settings. They are: (1) afterschool activities; (2) pastoral counseling and consultation; and (3) a bilingual CALACE[2] unit responsible for the advocacy of the service needs of the district's increasing Spanish-speaking populations. A fourth unit, the education unit, provides seminars and lectures to community organizations, to the C & E program, and to the center. The fifth unit, the research and evaluation unit, serves as an evaluation-support resource for the C & E program, the center, and programs within the community.

The units have the major responsibility for initiating new services when they are needed. These services are usually developed either by individual professional or paraprofessional unit members, or else by a subcommittee of a unit. The new service is then established within a new unit. The new services usually represent a mixture of staff interests, ongoing community needs, and responses to community crisis conditions (e.g., school desegregation).

The activities of each unit are summarized in the sections that follow. Each summary includes a description of unit activities carried out entirely or primarily by paraprofessionals. These activities often require competencies very different from those gained by professionals through formal education.

The afterschool unit is an example of a new service program designed to fill needs not currently being met within the catchment district. In this particular case, the public educational institutions were not always providing adequate social-emotional and institutional support to all of their constituents, particularly racial minorities and special-needs students; as a result, the needs of some children were not met by the existing programs. Three of the new services involving paraprofessionals (and professionals) are an afterschool tutorial and recreational program; programs to children within the school; and programs for parents. Parents are involved in all of these services, when possible, and in some instances the siblings of the child being served are also involved.

The pastoral unit focuses its efforts on helping pastors with counseling of parishioners and on offering a series of seminars to pastors on mental health issues (e.g. "crisis and communication in marriage and family life.") The unit also introduces pastors to the facilities and services of the center, helps the clergy to organize into action-oriented task forces, and involves churches in school desegregation efforts. The two members of this unit (a paraprofessional and a professional) share fully in all of the unit's activities.

[2]Comite de Asuntos Latino Americano de Consultoric y Education.

The CALACE unit is an example of a unit created in response to suggestions from staff members. Originally focusing on indirect and direct services to Spanish-speaking minorities, the members of this unit have recommended the creation of a transcultural committee to survey the needs of growing numbers of other non-English-speaking minorities in the catchment area.

Five of the seven unit members are paraprofessionals, and all members hold seats on relevant health and social agency boards. These affiliations have enabled the CALACE unit to organize a health task force, consisting of both the providers and the non-English-speaking consumers of health services. Paraprofessionals from the CALACE unit informed parents and students on school changes during the first year of school desegregation. The CALACE unit has also organized a referral network for Spanish-speaking residents. Collectively its members worked on a directory, "Latino Usame," a resource book for Hispanic consumers and non-Hispanic providers of human services in Boston.

The education unit is responsible for three broad activity areas: C & E in-service training, center in-service training, and community education. Paraprofessional staff members of the education unit supply a number of services. These services include educating both providers and consumers about existing and alternative community health delivery systems. Examples are lecture series to staff, training of school teachers, and a church-based series of seminars organized for consideration of problems faced by senior citizen enrollees.

The research and evaluation (R & E) unit gathers data, compiles reports, prepares forms, and involves staff members in program and self-evaluation efforts. It also serves the other mental health center programs as a central information source on (1) community resources and programs, and (2) the demography of the catchment area population served by the mental health center. This information is also made available to other community programs and has been extensively used by them in their own program planning.

In addition to its full-time staff, the unit also has a research and evaluation committee composed of a representative from each of the other units and from the two teams. This committee reviews and makes recommendations on recordkeeping and evaluation policy issues which affect the total C & E program.

The research and evaluation unit works closely with all the C & E teams. Each team is assigned an R & E paraprofessional who serves as a liaison with that team. This paraprofessional assists (1) in the maintenance of a cumulative information file on services the team is providing to the community programs with which it is working, and (2) in the creation and updating of a relevant community resource and directory file.

Unique Features.   The Fuller C & E program is characterized by two major features: (1) a community orientation, and (2) a complementary and equal-status relationship between the paraprofessional and the professional C & E staff members. This section describes how these features are put into practice.

A majority of the program's service personnel are technically mental health paraprofessionals, possessing a B.A. level degree or less (the nurse has an M.A.). The paraprofessionals are men and women who represent the major ethnic groups within the catchment district. The paraprofessionals feel that they have a good awareness of the community, and thus can act as community advocates whose ideas are relevant to community needs.

Each service staff member is assigned to a team by the program director. Furthermore, individuals acquire membership in one or more units according to interest and/or type of work they are doing. Unit leaders are appointed by the program director. These choices are based on the areas of specialization of staff members. The two team leaders and two coleaders are elected by the members of the given team independent of their professional status. Each team contains at least one member from every unit; furthermore, the members of each team are evenly distributed among the job categories created by the program's staffing grant. Both paraprofessional and professional staff members are quick to point out that team processes are very important in promoting the equal status relationships both between the paraprofessional and the professional staff members and among professionals from different disciplines. Within the teams the opinions of paraprofessionals and professionals are given equal weight. Furthermore, work plans depend on the special strengths, background, and skills of each team member.

One team is located in a residential brownstone or row house. This neighborhood residence is shared by the team and a community church. When not working in various community settings, team members spend most of their assignment time in the team offices. These offices are each crowded with three to six desks; as a consequence, team members can overhear conversations and can initiate informal and spontaneous interactions. The office arrangement, according to one staff paraprofessional, causes clients to identify the program staff with the community rather than with the center. (In contrast, the C & E floor at the center consists of isolated offices which face long corridors.)

One team leader describes his duties as consisting of "middle management by consensus." These duties include leading team meetings; preparing team reports; and taking or allocating responsibility for various team service, bookkeeping, purchasing, and bill-payment functions. The job is "not a position that one campaigns for"; the team leader receives no extra pay, and the role requires extra work. The leader is chosen on the basis of merit and popularity; the team must live with its choice for a subsequent period of time.

Team members report that they perform duties based on personal interest and competency rather than on degree level and/or discipline. The adjustment to this equal-status team arrangement, according to some staff members, may be more difficult for the professionals than for the paraprofessionals.

An emphasis on function also enhances the equal-status relationship of staff members outside of the teams. The new offices in the program's center location are assigned to units and also to individuals (whether professional or paraprofessional) who require the space for their duties. The program's few parking spaces are reserved for staff members who require space for two hours or less, thus enabling staff members to move between team and center locations.

Program Evaluation.   The program's evaluation specialists have gathered information on types of consultation (not education) offered by the C & E program and by the remaining programs in the center. Case consultation provides the major consultation focus (53% of total services) for non-C & E programs; this treatment-oriented function comprises the least prevalent consultative activity (13% of total services) in the C & E program. The C & E program's consultation activities focus predominantly on staff education (39%), program consultation (23%), and public information and education (25%); these nonclinical consultative services are considerably less common (47% of the total) in non-C & E programs.

Until recently the C & E program had not begun to develop and implement systematic program evaluation procedures. One exception to this policy occurred in the spring of 1973 when Ms. Ruth Batson, the first C & E Director, requested a questionnaire study to cover C & E services rendered between January 1 and October 1, 1973.[3] (Because of confidentiality considerations, this evaluation effort was limited to program-centered consultation.) Sixty-four organizations were contacted; the response rate was 83%.

The 1973 study of activities indicated a high (70–75%) rate of satisfaction with C & E services. It also showed that 91% of the consultees had heard of the C & E program prior to receiving services but that 76% of the service-oriented contacts were first made by the C & E staff.

In November 1976, the research and evaluation unit (of the C & E program) began to introduce more systematic recordkeeping procedures. The R & E unit by design contains at least one member from each C & E unit and a member from each team. Despite these staffing features, some six months of discussion were required before the final form of these revisions was agreed upon by the total C & E staff. The staff did not actively oppose recordkeeping; their attitude rather approximated a passive "Oh, my God, this as well!" The gradual introduction of change reflects the program's dedication to participatory decision making.

One feature of the recently revised evaluation procedures involves the community programs that receive continuing consultation from C & E staff members. When consultation is begun, the programs are now asked whether

[3]"Report on a Survey of User-Satisfaction with Consultative Services Offered by the Consultation and Education Program"—May 1974.

they are prepared to evaluate the consultation and the education services that they will receive. As soon as a termination-of-consultation report has been received from the C & E consultant, an evaluation questionnaire is now routinely sent to the consultee program to be returned directly to the C & E director and the R & E unit. (The option of sharing the evaluation judgment with the consultant is left with the party answering the questionnaire.) This procedure has the advantage of building in continuing consumer-satisfaction assessment; it is preferable to the cross-sectional approach represented by the previously described study conducted in 1973.

Use of Paraprofessionals

The term "paraprofessional" is not commonly used by the program staff members, nor are other types of distinctions made between paraprofessionals and professionals. The staff members interviewed reported performing functions related to their skills and interests rather than being restricted by their levels of formal education. Distinctions reflecting degree level, however, are applied to the program by the state of Massachusetts. The state makes three basic distinctions: professional (M.A. or above); B.A. level; and sub-B.A. level.

The paraprofessional-professional distinction was also very important to Dr. Bernard Bandler when he initiated the C & E program. It was Dr. Bandler's belief that a "critical mass" of paraprofessionals was necessary to create and maintain a program's community orientation.

The paraprofessional staff members are essential to the functioning of the C & E program. Their skills are particularly appropriate in the area of community advocacy. They are the agents who forge the links between the center (as well as the C & E program) and the community. The paraprofessionals supplement these general community-related functions with more specialized skills. When interviewed, staff members reported that the skills and responsibilities of paraprofessionals far exceed the state job descriptions. Characteristically, the paraprofessionals have voluntarily upgraded their skills through challenging, self-chosen work and formal training experiences.

The paraprofessionals choose or even design their work activities within the framework of the team's perception of and response to community mental health needs. As illustrated in the following paragraphs, each paraprofessional can express personal interests and pursue individual goals through work.

One black male paraprofessional combines an interest in students, mental health education, and photography. He has developed a drug education program for teenagers that makes liberal use of slides and tapes, and has created a high school course on mental health. He works with the school desegregation crisis team and has helped to establish an afterschool program for high school students being bused.

A Spanish-speaking female paraprofessional enjoys outreach, coordination, and consultation functions. She currently is a community worker, the coordinator of the CALACE Unit, and a consultant to professionals and nonprofessionals from varying disciplines and backgrounds. She visits various organizations within the catchment district, focusing especially on groups that serve Spanish-speaking clients. Her first task is to establish a relationship and to explain the functions of the C & E program to the organization. Then she asks the group to describe its concerns and problems. And, finally, she helps the organization to secure the relevant consultation or education services from the program. When she feels it is appropriate, she provides consultation services to the group. The C & E program has provided her with her first work-based opportunity for realization of her long-time personal goal, to go to college. By completing her A.A., working on her B.A., and continuing her career, she has overcome a cultural tradition that disapproves of these activities by a married woman with children.

A third example of paraprofessional accomplishment is provided by a black woman who specializes in administrative functions and children's services. Her duties include being one of the program's two team leaders, serving as the "right-hand person" to the program director, representing the program on the State Drug Advisory Board, and teaching seminars on developmental problems to day care instructors. She was hired as a high school graduate, but has since earned an A.A. degree and will soon complete her B.A. She has carried out her educational activities while continuing to work full time.

Difficulties occasionally arise in a C & E program. The types of problems that are described immediately following represent generalizations from the interviews with program staff members. It is important to note that not all interviewees agree on the existence of all problems.

Some paraprofessionals report that certain professionals, both in the community and in other center programs, do not treat paraprofessionals with the same respect as staff members with advanced degrees. In some cases these attitudes do not change with time, but often the professionals revise their opinions after working with competent, skilled paraprofessionals.

People in the community also seem at times to question the competence of paraprofessionals. Not infrequently, especially with regard to testing, community organizations specifically request professionals for C & E services. Program staff members do not always agree with the appropriateness of the agency's request for a professional. It is sometimes useful to send paraprofessionals and professionals in pairs on agency assignments, with the paraprofessional assuming equal or major responsibility for service delivery.

In the C & E program in Boston, paraprofessionals occasionally deliver direct services, even though assigned to deliver only indirect services. When faced with a concrete direct service need, it is sometimes difficult for paraprofessionals not to respond. On occasion an organization that has requested the assistance of a paraprofessional from the C & E program will ask the paraprofessional to perform direct service functions. A staff member suggested two possible solutions to this problem: (1) training paraprofessionals to understand the value of C & E services, and how, by teaching their skills to others, they accomplish much more than by doing direct services themselves; and (2) making sure that paraprofessionals are able to say "no" to requests for direct services, perhaps through assertiveness training or role playing.

Some interviewees state that paraprofessionals do not appreciate the value of theory and academic knowledge, as opposed to information concerning specific practices and situations. This attitude may reflect a reaction to excessive use of jargon and abstractions among professionals. There also seems to be some resistance by paraprofessionals to recordkeeping and evaluation, and to supervision even when it may be helpful or necessary. These mechanisms provide paraprofessionals with systematic, ongoing feedback so that they do not overestimate or underestimate their skills.

Recruitment

The program usually does not actively recruit staff paraprofessionals; rather, potential candidates hear about the C & E program informally and then seek employment. The C & E paraprofessionals at Fuller report being attracted to the program's work situation, to the work content, and/or to salary and job security features.

Selection

A two-committee (community and professional) selection procedure was abandoned after the original C & E staff was hired. Currently, prospective employees (both professional and paraprofessional) are screened by a committee of six C & E staff members (five paraprofessionals, one R.N.). Four of the members of this committee are female; the committee is balanced ethnically. When a professional person applies, the committee is supplemented by a professional staff member from the given candidate's field. The equal-status working conditions are emphasized to professionals. The committee recommends to the director of the program three candidates for each position. The director then chooses the new employee from the three unranked candidates. Staff members uniformly report the absence of sex or racial discrimination in the program.

In general, the members of the interview committee look for paraprofessionals who exhibit a potential and a desire for growth, the ability to be flexible and independent at work, and a capacity for successful interactions with professional staff members. Interest and energy are other valued personal qualities. Most staff paraprofessionals have engaged in related paid work experience, volunteer work, or training prior to employment.

Training

All staff members (professional or paraprofessional) are expected to attend in-service seminars and workshops. This formal training, however, is supplemented by informal learning in the context of the teams—group job assignments, team meetings, and informal discussions. Currently, the educational unit is developing plans for a more systematic orientation and in-service training program.

At present a staff member is developing a formal orientation manual for new employees. The plan is for new employees to learn skills and gain perspective on the program's activities through a "buddy" system. Initially, new employees will spend considerable time with a team, observing the program's activities first hand. As they gain a perspective on the scope of the program, they will spend a greater proportion of time in unit activities. At the end of two months, new employees will choose an area of specialization.

Supervision

Supervision within the program is largely spontaneous and informal, rather than planned and structured. And the supervision that exists is two-way in nature; professionals and paraprofessionals learn from each other.

The chief mechanism for supervision has been described by one papaprofessional staff member as more closely approximating "peer counseling." Staff members feel free to ask other staff members for assistance. This assistance is generally requested spontaneously (but it can be arranged on a regular basis); the assistance is nonjudgmental, resembling the interchanges of friends. The peer counseling can involve information exchange, the expression of emotions, and the exploration of alternatives for action. Individuals who do not request these informal conferences do not receive this form of supervision.

The team structure provides a vehicle for much supervision since many informal information-laden conversations occur in team offices and meetings. Furthermore, the teams send interdisciplinary groups appropriate to the given situation out on community assignments, where paraprofessionals and professionals can learn from one another by working together on the same assignments.

There are particular attitudes and skills that paraprofessional staff members feel they can offer professional staff. These include: (1) processes for contacting and communicating with community citizens and agencies; (2) alternatives to unnecessary professional jargon; (3) respect for community people; (4) knowledge about the community, including awareness of community needs; and (5) awareness (in specific cases) that behavior reflects cultural and adaptive traits rather than psychopathology.

Mobility

Because of the state civil service restrictions, the program cannot offer a degree-independent career ladder to paraprofessional staff members. Sub-B.A. people are restricted to one step in possible promotions, and B.A. level staff members are restricted to four steps. Promotions are based on skill and length of service, as well as on the earning of a higher degree. The hiring committee recommends promotions within the state limits, contingent on the availability of a slot to be filled. The program tries to offset career ladder restrictions by being flexible in arranging time off for sub-B.A. staff members *working towards a degree.* Staff members occasionally accumulate vacation time to attend special school programs (at Goddard University and Antioch College) geared for B.A. or M.A. candidates who work full time.

Although the C & E paraprofessionals feel that they are underpaid in comparison to program professionals, the current turnover rate for paraprofessionals is low. Most people who have left the C & E program during the past six months have been staff members who either received a more responsible position elsewhere or wanted to attend an educational program on a full-time basis.

A few of the program's professionals (as well as a previous C & E director) are former paraprofessional service workers who have earned higher degrees after beginning to work with the program. These staff people demonstrate that paraprofessionals can gain professional credentials. This outcome is not surprising, since the hiring process selects upwardly mobile paraprofessionals.

Status and Morale

One of the most striking features of the C & E program at the Fuller Center is the high morale of the staff. These positive feelings exist despite paraprofessionals' dissatisfaction with salaries.

Salary. The paraprofessionals uniformly describe their salaries as being too low for the responsibilities they carry out and as inadequate to support a family. They perceive their job responsibilities as being equivalent to those executed by professionals. Some dissatisfaction is also expressed at the lack of opportunity for promotion of sub-B.A. staff members. Two paraprofessionals say that they would execute more complex and demanding tasks if they were given higher salaries. But paraprofessionals uniformly blame these perceived inequities on the state job classification system.

Interpersonal Relations. Paraprofessional and professional staff alike report good relationships with professionals, paraprofessionals, and the program director. (One or two professionals are resented by some paraprofessionals for not appearing to work hard enough for the salaries received.) Staff members feel respected for their individual talents. Paraprofessionals report that most professionals do not hold elitist attitudes and attribute the good interpersonal relationships to several factors: (1) the open communication processes initiated by Ms. Batson and continued by Ms. Garcia; (2) the family-like atmosphere in teams; and (3) the fact that professionals and paraprofessionals collaborate on a number of projects.

Satisfaction with Individual Work Responsibilities.   Paraprofessionals uniformly report satisfaction with their levels of work responsibility. They
enjoy the opportunities for initiating new program activities, providing input
to various ongoing program activities, and carrying out a wide and varying
assortment of work duties.

Staff members report several additional positive features of the program.
They state that they freely seek advice and express feelings within teams, units,
and other settings—staff members, thus, serve as peer advisors to one another.
Teams decide collectively who will communicate important "gripes" to the
program director, and these complaints are conveyed openly and frankly.
Important policy changes within the C & E program are generally implemented *slowly* and in consultation with the entire program staff, and initiative
by all staff members is encouraged and accepted. For example, a paraprofessional is developing, through the afterschool unit, a series of photographs and
slides to be used in a program for adolescents, and a subcommittee of the
education unit is developing a C & E staff orientation manual to be used by
members of the education unit. The program often has group recreational
activities, ranging from a volleyball game to a money-raising bazaar for a
community project. These group activities seem to play an important role in
promoting the equal-status relationships and group solidarity that are hall-
marks of the Fuller C & E program.

Evaluation of Paraprofessional Performance

Performance evaluation procedures (until recently) have been nonsystematic;
much evaluation occurs informally during team meetings. Additional evaluation occurs through informal feedback (e.g., attendance rates in a seminar)
from community organizations or clients. The introduction of goal-related
evaluation procedures is difficult in the context of the indirect nature of the
program's services and its tradition of trusting individuals to perform competently.

Two procedures introduced recently require staff self-evaluation. One
recordkeeping form—completed when a client contact is initiated—requires
the C & E staff members to list their goals in the order of priority. Furthermore, as deliverers of mental health services, the staff person must describe the
source of initiation (agency, staff member, or some mix) of each given goal.
At the termination of each contact, the staff member discusses in a second form
the specific goals that were and were not completely accomplished.

In Conclusion

The C & E program serves as a bridge between the community and the Dr.
Solomon Carter Fuller Community Mental Health Center. It enables the
center to provide more relevant services to the community, and also helps the

community to educate the center about its needs. In addition, the C & E program performs the traditional C & E services.

C & E paraprofessionals play critical roles in making possible the implementation of all program functions. As representatives of the community, the paraprofessionals assist in establishing liaisons with the community and in teaching both C & E and other center professionals about the community. The fact that the paraprofessionals are indigenous, however, accounts only in part for their impact; structural features of the C & E program are critical. A significant proportion of C & E staff members are paraprofessionals, comprising a "critical mass" with a group identity. Both directors of the C & E program are indigenous paraprofessionals. Paraprofessionals and professionals work together on an equal-status basis in community-based team settings, and, within competency-based limits, participate fully in the design and delivery of the services offered by the C & E program.

Chapter 6

DAY CARE AND OTHER PARTIAL
HOSPITALIZATION SERVICES

INTRODUCTION

Description of the Service Area

The provision of day care and other partial hospitalization services is one of the areas of service delivery that was newly mandated by the 1975 Community Mental Health Center Amendments. This legislation requires that a community mental health center provides individualized therapeutic and rehabilitative services for those persons who require less than 24-hour care but more than outpatient care. This type of treatment has proved to be an effective alternative to inpatient care and has emerged as the treatment of choice for many persons previously thought to require full-time care. Since patients are at the mental health center only part of the time, they continue to participate in the life of the community. They may work, attend school, or simply spend time with their families.

Day care can also serve as a transition between full-time care and the individual's return to the community. This allows for an appreciable shortening of a person's inpatient stay. Services intended for this purpose should be designed not only to treat mental health problems, but also to improve basic coping, social, and vocational skills which are necessary for successful community functioning. Such services should be provided in a nonmedical "normalizing" milieu, minimizing labeling and dependency and providing opportunities for clients to assume responsible problem-solving roles.

Program content and schedules for day care should reflect an assessment of the needs and resources within the catchment area, and must provide not less than a half-day program five days a week, as well as care for other periods. Various alternative partial care programs might include overnight inpatient stays, a weekend program, or an evening program. These variations in program scheduling would be offered to encourage clients to maintain or reestablish typical living patterns involving work, school, and family life. In addition, the potential for involvement of family in the treatment process is increased.

Partial hospitalization services should be tailored to meet the needs of special categories of clients, for example, drug abusers, alcoholics, adolescents, chronically disabled adults, and elderly persons. Some centers may find such specialization necessary to meet community needs whereas in other instances such a formal subdivision of services may be unnecessary or undesirable. In any case, innovative arrangements are encouraged as long as they are consistent with sound mental health practices.

In addition to the following case study, the interested reader may wish to refer to the chapters covering transitional services and follow-up services, which contain descriptions of programs which overlap somewhat with this service area.

Selection of the Site Visited

Psychosocial rehabilitation programs provide, through a noninstitutional-type setting or "club," vocational, social-residential, recreational, and evaluative services. These programs build on the strengths of clients, who assist staff members in the actual operation of the program. The psychosocial rehabilitation model provides services mandated by National Institute of Mental Health guidelines for the day care and other partial hospitalization service area.

NIMH has recently expressed a particular concern for chronic patients, that is, people who are seriously disabled by long-term mental problems. One of the architects of the Community Support System, Judy Turner of the Mental Health Services Support Branch of NIMH, recommended that we examine the ways paraprofessionals are used in psychosocial rehabilitation programs to assist these clients.

The Club, a program of the Community Mental Health Center of the Rutgers Medical School, has integrated the psychosocial rehabilitation model into the operations of a large mental health center. The Club employs a high ratio of paraprofessionals and trains them in specific skills to serve an often neglected client population. Since we were particularly interested in service delivery models that make extensive and effective use of paraprofessionals, this led to our choice of The Club as appropriate for a site visit.

The Club: A Case Study in Day Care and Other Partial Hospitalization Services*

The Club is a psychosocial rehabilitation program located within a wing of the Community Mental Health Center of the Rutgers Medical School. The Club provides a variety of social, vocational, educational, residential, and evaluative services to clients who are considered club members rather than patients. This chapter describes The Club as an example of day care and partial hospitalization services.

The center is located on the outskirts of Piscataway, New Jersey, and its personnel emphasize services to youth and to families. The active case load of about 3,500 clients is drawn mostly from working class white people who live in small towns throughout the catchment area. The center also serves urban New Brunswick, a town that contains a more ethnically varied population, as well as the students of Rutgers University. Besides the large mental health center adjoining the medical school complex, there are four community focus teams which operate from satellite centers.

Background

The center was started in 1972 in order to provide research and teaching opportunities for the medical school and mental services for the community. From its inception, the mental health center's executive director and chairman of the Department of Psychiatry, Dr. Irwin Pollack, wanted to provide good aftercare and rehabilitation services to the center clientele. In 1973, the Rutgers Community Mental Health Center hired Mr. Julius Lanoil to develop a psychosocial rehabilitation program. Soon after Mr. Lanoil was hired, he received a grant from the social rehabilitation services of the Department of Health, Education, and Welfare which permitted him to hire three staff members. Mr. Lanoil came to Rutgers with eight years of experience at Fountain House Foundation. Fountain House is a psychosocial rehabilitation center located in a large, attractive, Georgian colonial building in the Hell's Kitchen section of New York City. It was here that pioneer work in the area of psychosocial rehabilitation for ex-mental patients took place. Lanoil took many of the concepts from Fountain House and applied them to the community mental health center setting. By 1976, The Club in Piscataway had almost 200 active members (attending at least once a month). The staff now consists of 15 paid workers and about 60 volunteers. The vast majority have a B.A.

*Contact: The Community Mental Health Center of the Rutgers Medical School
         P. O. Box 101
         Piscataway, New Jersey   08854
         201/564-4375
         Attention: Julius Lanoil, Director, Habilitation Service

degree or less, thus emphasizing the importance of paraprofessional staff members at The Club.

Considering the unique responsibilities of staff members at The Club, to be described in detail later in this chapter, a new job slot called "habilitation counselor" was created for these primarily paraprofessional Club employees. The term *re*habilitation implies that clients are being returned to a previously achieved level of competence. In general, the clients at The Club have never achieved an adequate level of socialization and thus workers must try to "habilitate" them. Habilitation workers earn from $11,365 to $13,157 per year, with supervising habilitation counselors earning $15,321.

Theoretical Underpinnings.   The professional and nonprofessional staff members at The Club share a commitment to the frequently discussed philosophy of The Club. Besides the weekly staff meeting where practical problems are dealt with, there is another weekly meeting for discussion of more theoretical issues such as "What about dependency of clients?"; "Seduction and persuasion as methods of motivating members"; "The role of work in the rehabilitation process"; and so on. The staff believe that an action or decision that would compromise The Club's theoretical underpinnings should be avoided, even if it has short-term advantages.

One of the ideas which is crucial to The Club's approach is that of mutual interdependence of staff and members. The habilitation workers are not there to serve the clients. Such an approach, according to The Club philosophy, would encourage passivity and retard growth. By intent and structure, the workers at The Club genuinely need the members to do things, because the programs cannot be maintained without their active participation. A new member can easily see that the kitchen is understaffed or that someone is needed to answer the phone. The focus of the worker is on what the member *can do,* on his or her competencies. Club staff members feel that all too often traditional mental health personnel only pay attention to the clients' problems and illness. Even staff in other parts of the mental health center will sometimes express surprise at seeing one of their patients, still hallucinating perhaps, working adequately, if not efficiently, at the snack bar. All the common interaction patterns that go on between people, such as praise, arguments, disappointments, rewards, punishments, and expectations, also go on between The Club staff and the members. Interactions are public and nonsecluded. Workers are encouraged to express their feelings if they feel manipulated, angry, or pleased by their relationship with a Club member. As Lanoil puts it, "Interactions are nonritualistic." Workers are not expected to fall back on professional roles for their authority. Instead, they must exert their personalities to function as naturally evolved leaders in the community. The Club philosophy maintains that it is important to frame the relationships between workers and members in the context of mutual interdependence. The staff workers need the members to help complete tasks for which they are responsible. The members need the workers to assist them in the practical problems of living: finding a place to live, finding a job, and working out conflicts with friends.

In contrast with some other psychosocial rehabilitation programs, The Club places no time limits on how long a client may participate in its activities. A person's move from dependence to independence is an individual process. Some members may never be totally independent. The Club provides a social network of habilitation workers and other clients who actively reach out to establish relationships. There is a great deal of continuity in the members' involvement with The Club. They get to know other members and workers even before they are released from the state hospital. The habilitation worker assigned to work with the member will continue that relationship as long as the member belongs to The Club. The same staff member may work alongside a member making curtains, train the member to work in a fast food chain, help arrange for an apartment, assist in painting and decorating the apartment, take the member bowling, and share a Christmas dinner. As individual members establish their own group of friends or positive relations with their own family, they need the center less; but members always have the option to drop by The Club and to visit.

Julius Lanoil likes to quote Mr. John Beard, Executive Director of Fountain House, in explaining the work of The Club as the building of "invisible social ramps or prosthetic devices. As in physical rehabilitation, mechanical aids are developed which permit a person who is disabled to function as if he were not disabled. If a person has no legs, one can create artificial legs, fit them, and teach the person to walk on them. In the area of psychiatric rehabilitation, the ramps or prosthetic devices must be invisible but nonetheless very real, since they involve interpersonal relationships and the supports that the patient feels as a result." The Club attempts to develop these invisible ramps and prosthetic devices which permit a person to work, to live independently, to go to school, and to participate in recreational activities.

Program Organization and Services

The program is aimed at meeting the needs of a generally neglected population, chronically hospitalized people, who although they do not presently require intensive psychiatric treatment, do need extensive support to help them live outside an institution. Most of the clients lack the skills required for coping with the day-to-day world, such as renting and furnishing an apartment, finding and keeping a job, and finding friends and recreational opportunities. The Club aims at developing a community support system for individuals discharged from hospitals or for those people who might be able to avoid hospitalization with such assistance. The facilities at The Club are comfortable and brightly painted. The music areas, snack bar, sewing rooms, and other areas are designed to suggest a nonclinical setting. The Club is open five days and two evenings per week and for at least half a day on all holidays. Most of the members are recruited while they are still in the nearby state hospital; however, clients might be referred directly to The Club by someone from another agency. Staff and Club members visit the hospital once a week, talk to patients who are from the center catchment area, explain the program, and invite those people who seem able to leave the hospital to be Club members. While they are still patients, prospective members can leave the hospital in one of The Club vans to visit The Club for the day. Such visits usually increase in frequency as the time for the patient's discharge approaches.

Members of The Club can participate in a number of activities: prevocational day program, work-for-pay program, social recreation, and special programs. Each of these will be discussed separately, but the separation is only conceptual. Clients and staff members overlap among all the programs and there is a deliberate attempt to avoid specialization. Continuity of care is considered important and is created primarily by the continuity of the member's relationship with a specific staff person through many Club activities.

Prevocational Day Care.   Club members who are felt to need "day care" and others who merely enjoy the social milieu spend the day at The Club. Some drop in; others are picked up at their residences by Club vans and are brought to the center. Some of The Club members who have cars and work as drivers are volunteers and they are reimbursed for car expenses by the center. In addition, there are other members who have been hired by The Club to drive vans for which they are paid the normal rate for such positions. Each habilitation worker is involved in a specific activity area which is necessary for the maintenance and growth of The Club. For example, one worker is in charge of the dining room area; another handles custodial tasks. Club members are not "treated" when they come to The Club; instead, the habilitation worker attempts to involve the member in helping the worker fulfill his or her responsibilities. Thus, the worker in charge of the dining room must involve Club members in the preparation and serving of the daily lunch (sold for a bargain price of 60 cents, which is partially subsidized by the Mental Health Center). The Club philosophy states that every member has something to contribute and staff members draw on the members' capacities and strengths. The Club does not use the regular janitorial services of the mental health center but depends on its own members to assist the habilitation workers to maintain and decorate the space it uses. Another example of cooperation between workers and members is the clerical program. Participants collect and collate attendance and other forms of data on The Club, publish a weekly newspaper and a monthly magazine, and provide switchboard coverage. In addition, there is a garden, a plant shop, a sewing room, and a woodworking shop at The Club.

Some members run tours for visitors. Others are assigned to reach out to members who are, for emotional reasons, homebound. Their task is to attempt to convince them to attend Club activities. In addition, all clients who return to a psychiatric hospital are visited by members and workers and receive weekly and monthly publications. In all these activities, members assist in the tasks of maintaining their Club. The process of interacting with other members and workers in organizing and following through on tasks and taking on responsibility is considered useful in preparing members to move toward paid employment and increased independence.

Members who come to the center may discuss problems with their habilitation worker, but the emphasis is on the here and now. The practical problems of relationships with other Club or staff members or of work problems are emphasized, rather than what is traditionally considered psychotherapy. No group therapy sessions are scheduled although, in the course of a joint work task, personal and interpersonal problems are sometimes discussed. Some of the members are in individual therapy with their own therapists or a therapist from another part of the center.

In general, the day care component of The Club provides a pleasant supportive environment where members are encouraged to participate in the active and ongoing work of The Club.

Work-for-Pay Program. The work-for-pay program deals with employment at the mental health center as well as transitional employment. A number of members are employed by the mental health center or the associated medical school on an occasional or regular basis and receive the regular rate of pay for that job. These jobs include maintenance, clerical work, and assistance in transporting persons from the center to a psychiatric hospital. Persons who are too anxious and upset to accept a job in the community may be willing to work in the more familiar environment of the medical school complex.

The habilitation workers work closely with the job supervisors to assist in on-the-job problems. Club members are paid by the medical school units they work for, although, if a unit needs help but does not have funds in its budget, the mental health center may assign The Club to fill the need and subsidize the medical school unit to pay The Club member. The employment program provides an opportunity for the medical school community to become involved in the rehabilitation of former mental patients. The jobs in which members are hired typically have a high turnover rate. Placement of Club members in these positions, backed up by habilitation workers, helps to ensure that these jobs are always filled.

The transitional employment program places members in actual work situations in community businesses. At present The Club has 12 part-time placements with five different businesses in the community. There are permanent placements in such businesses as restaurants, warehouses, and grocery stores. The Club selects a member for an employee position when The Club staff believes that the member can handle a job with some Club support. The transitional employment program is not considered so much a vocational training program as an opportunity for members to test their current ability to work in a real job.

The Club member is interviewed by the employer and, if hired, is paid at the regular job rate. Members work in these jobs on a half-time basis for three or four months. Then they are rotated to another job and new members replace them. The employer only has to perform job training with one individual, a habilitation worker from The Club. Then the habilitation worker trains Club members to do the job, and if The Club member is unable to work, the habilitation worker fills in temporarily. In this way, the employer does not need to undertake training of every Club member entering employment, and job coverage is guaranteed. In high turnover, semiskilled jobs, these factors are appealing to employers. The Club member is expected to perform as well as any other employee, and the habilitation workers check with the supervisor to make sure that the member receives honest feedback on job performance and has the opportunity to experience the demands of a real job in the community.

Recreational Activities.   No traditional recreational therapy activities are scheduled at The Club, but a wide variety of activities such as dinners, dramatics, photography, craft groups, trips to local theaters, and sports activities take place in the evenings, and on weekends and holidays. Since holidays are often a time of stress for members, events such as a New Year's Eve party and Christmas and Thanksgiving dinners are particularly important. The Club sees itself as establishing a social network of relationships for members who often have poor family relations and no friends.

Special Projects.   The special projects program of The Club includes a learning opportunities program, a beauty parlor, a barber shop, vocational counseling, and a social skills training group. The learning opportunities program links a community volunteer with one or two Club members for mutual study in an area of mutual interest. All Club members are given some sort of education evaluation, either formal or informal, by the learning opportunities coordinator, who has a B.A. degree in education. This evaluation enables the coordinator to identify the educational interests and needs of the members. Some club members need basic literacy skills. Others have interests in topics as diverse as poetry, mechanics, or cooking. Volunteers who participate in the learning opportunities program are carefully screened and helped to improve their teaching skills. They participate in a 10-hour preservice program and meet with The Club staff members once every three weeks in an in-service training program. Most of the tutors are college students who receive college credit for tutoring. While they are enthusiastic volunteers, college students are a transient population and usually move on to a new community or a new interest after a semester or two. The learning opportunities coordinator is committed to the ideals of self-help and would prefer to move The Club in the direction of peer tutoring rather than continuing to rely on volunteers from the community. He believes that traditional adult education programs do not meet the needs of chronically hospitalized clients who need the security of small group or individual work in a supportive atmosphere. It is also felt that the educational process can be an important tool in the rehabilitation of ex-patients. The coordinator cited the case of a severely isolated woman who, with the help of tutoring, was able to pass her written test for a driver's license and thus use the family car to increase her social contacts.

Other special projects include the participation of an employee of the State Division of Vocational Rehabilitation who works with staff members in vocational counseling and evaluation of clients for job training. A volunteer barber comes in twice weekly to cut men's hair and tutor some of the men in barbering. A beauty shop has been set up where women members help each other to wash and set hair.

Residential Programs.   The Club has available two types of residential programs. One is an 18-bed halfway house in The Club, next door to the center's inpatient unit. This short-term residential program is designed for those members who have just recently left an inpatient facility. It is also used to prevent rehospitalization of those members who, for a time, need the close support the halfway house offers. The halfway house is a nonmedical facility. The residents receive medication and supportive psychiatric treatment from two other mental health center programs—either the New Brunswick Community Focus Team or Acute Psychiatric Services.

The comfortable dormlike living area is located directly upstairs from The Club, providing easy access for both Club members and staff personnel. Originally, habilitation workers lived in the halfway house with the members. Later, more mature Club members took over the responsibility for the area, living there rent-free. Staff members plan trips on all weekends and holidays. At the present time, habilitation counselors and college student volunteers take shifts supervising the area. The members in the program prepare their own meals, clean the facilities, and participate in the Club activities downstairs. Each member pays a rental fee of $20 per week.

The second residential program is called SERV. It grew out of the desire by Club members to get their own apartments. The members were usually inexperienced in independent living and often lacked the funds necessary to pay for the security deposit on an apartment and to buy furniture for it. The Club staff members devised a plan in which The Club would lease apartments from landlords and then sublease them to members. Because The Club is administered by the state, there were legal complications in providing this service through The Club. Instead, a nonprofit organization called SERV Centers of New Jersey, Inc., was developed. While it is a financially separate entity, the original staff members were previously Club habilitation workers and its activities are closely linked to The Club. SERV not only subleases the apartments to 57 members, but helps them to decorate, assists them in grocery shopping, and helps them to learn skills in activities of daily living, such as cooking and personal hygiene. Each apartment has a habilitation worker assigned to it. Clusters of apartments within the same complex have weekly meetings and the members plan recreational and shopping trips together. In a typical situation, several Club members will share an apartment. On occasion, habilitation workers help the roommates work out personal differences. SERV also functions in the role of tenant advocate, assisting the tenant in obtaining needed repairs or handling landlord-tenant conflicts. The SERV program is advantageous to the landlord who is guaranteed rent from a responsible group, who does not have to locate new tenants if the apartment is vacated, and who has a SERV staff member who will assist in dealing with problems such as tenant damage.

In the first year of the program, two SERV staff members lived in a SERV apartment within a cluster of SERV apartments. They were not seen as staff members on duty, but rather as neighbors who could be called on for help. Their presence was also reassuring to the landlords. As SERV starts its second year, members have been accepted as tenants by the landlord, who no longer needs the reassurance of having a staff member on site to solve problems. Thus, the staff members are moving out and The Club members will be expected to support each other.

Use of Paraprofessionals

The field of psychosocial rehabilitation is a new one, and it seems particularly well-suited to the use of paraprofessional personnel. Across the United States there are currently about 200 centers with differing approaches to the field. The centers attempt to meet a wide range of client needs: economic, housing, transportation, recreation, social, and to develop social networks to support the client in making a life outside of an institution. Traditional psychological, psychiatric, or social work training does not prepare individuals to work with chronic clients in this way. Even professional staff members in a psychosocial rehabilitation program do not necessarily have this background and must often be trained in new concepts and skills. The advantage of the professional staff member's prior training, therefore, carries little weight for psychosocial programs. Indeed, because paraprofessionals have not been trained in an alternative approach, they are sometimes more open to learn the concepts and skills of psychosocial rehabilitation.

Paraprofessionals are also ideal staff members for programs such as The Club because they are generally more willing to take on difficult and often unglamorous tasks which professionals might consider "unprofessional." A habilitation counselor might wash dishes along with a client, run a literary magazine, or help arrange canned goods on the shelves of a client's new apartment. Thus, the staff person must come to understand the reasons for the kinds of approaches used and how they relate to the rehabilitation of the schizophrenic.

The Club has had few problems in using paraprofessional personnel. Lanoil stresses the importance of establishing good relations between the staff members of the psychosocial rehabilitation program and the staff members of the other parts of the community mental health center. Clinicians need to be educated about the program and the role of the habilitation workers. The noncredentialed workers may be intimidated by the clinicians or physicians unless these professionals are educated about the theory of psychosocial rehabilitation and unless the workers see themselves as "experts."

The large numbers and diverse kinds of demands faced daily put a great deal of stress on the workers. There is a tendency to "burn out." The Club has attempted to deal with this problem by providing a great deal of peer support, by shifting work roles frequently, and by rallying staff members around a commitment to the principles in which they believe.

Recruitment

Since few job openings occur at The Club, recruitment of personnel has been casual. Some employees came to The Club as student volunteers, one was a CETA worker, others came to the hospital looking for a position. One counselor was a Club member who showed his ability by his work and finally was hired.

Selection

In the selection process, Lanoil says that they look for "hungry people" eager to do things. Often these individuals have been frustrated by the formal education system, or they have had life experiences that caused them to understand what it is to suffer and then to arrive at a solution. Prospective habilitation workers must be able to feel comfortable with people whose behavior is often deviant. Interviews do not seem to be as successful in screening good workers as having them come to visit the center for a day to participate in the daily activities. After working in the snack bar, talking with members, and getting to know other staff, both the prospective employee and the staff members have a better sense of whether or not the candidate should be hired.

When looking for Club staff, personal characteristics are considered more important than degrees. Two of the habilitation counselors have M.A. degrees but this was not (and is not) a requirement for the job. Prospective employees must agree with the therapeutic goals and methods involved in the psychosocial program and philosophy. They must be able to adjust their self-image to the kinds of activities required of them and they must find the program consistent with their abilities and predilections for therapeutic involvement.

Lanoil believes that staff members must have personal charisma. The emotional intensity of the relationship between the habilitation counselor and The Club member is important in eliciting the involvement of the members. This relationship also encourages the member to act in nonpsychotic ways, congruent with the behavior norm established by the counselor and The Club.

Training

While there is some basic orientation given to new staff members, most training seems to take place on the job as the new staff member works alongside an older staff person in an apprentice-like situation. New employees must take responsibility quickly. When the first group of staff members were hired, they had long discussions, often lasting late into the night, at a counselor's home, talking over the ideas of psychosocial rehabilitation. There are now weekly sessions to discuss concepts in psychosocial rehabilitation and these are seen as an important part of in-service training. Most training comes on the job, with peers and supervisory staff members giving feedback on the spot. While the counselors have a great deal of responsibility, they are expected to ask for assistance when they need it. A climate of openness and trust is important for this to happen. A general concern in the field of mental health is the question of whether paraprofessional staff have sufficient training to work with individuals with severe mental problems. Habilitation workers do not treat the clients therapeutically. While the workers may help the member deal with a specific problem such as work, transportation, or housing, the workers do not probe into the members' past or psychological problems. In response to criticisms that paraprofessionals do not have the sophisticated diagnostic skills required to assess the client's mental status, The Club psychiatrist points out that the workers spend a massive amount of time interacting with most members. This enables them to be sensitive to the changes in the members' behavior and moods without the highly sophisticated training that might be necessary if the client was seen only periodically for a short time.

Supervision

Habilitation counselors are divided into two teams. The team leaders supervise their staff by reading case notes, reviewing specific cases in weekly team meetings, and by on-the-spot feedback. The staff members seem unusually open to suggestions and criticisms from their peers and even from members. The project director position is held by a woman who has not completed her B.A. degree. Some of the staff she supervises have M.A.s. While some centers have reported problems having paraprofessionals supervise those with higher academic degrees, The Club has not had such difficulties. Perhaps the lack of strong identification with one's specific profession, along with strong commitment to the common ideals of The Club, make this an easier situation.

Career Mobility

Lanoil believes that the field of psychosocial rehabilitation is a good one for paraprofessionals since they are offering important and unique services not provided by any professional group. Furthermore, most professionals find the population of undermotivated chronic schizophrenics who have a long history of hospitalization a difficult and unrewarding group with which to work. He envisions the expansion of the field with trained workers initiating and staffing other programs.

A new habilitation counselor series was developed for Club employees in the community mental health center. While this classification system raises the amount of money that can be earned, the size of The Club program and lack of turnover limits much upward mobility within the Club structure. After four years of working in the program, a woman with a B.A. degree was given the job of program director. She was selected because of her interest and competence in administrative work. Most workers believe that they can become team leaders without an M.A. degree, but consider an advanced degree necessary for upward mobility if they move outside The Club.

Education

The in-service program is not accredited for work toward a B.A. or M.A. degree. A local college does give undergraduate field experience credit for a placement at The Club. While individual staff members have been able to arrange time off to take courses, making up the time on other occasions, this has not been a satisfactory process primarily because the daily demands of the job are so great that it is difficult both physically and psychologically to get away.

Lanoil is currently designing a curriculum for a B.A. and M.A. in the field of psychosocial rehabilitation to meet what he sees as the growing need for training in this area. The program would involve a mixture of coursework, independent study, and fieldwork.

Status and Morale

The habilitation workers reported that they feel very positive about the work they are doing. They obtain satisfaction from the relationships they have with other staff and from their relationships with Club members. The workers report that morale is high and that they have a sense of doing something worthwhile and being committed to an important principle. They are respected by the other staff members at the mental health center. Their relationships with clients are generally quite positive. On a typical walk around The Club, however, one might find a client arguing vigorously with a habilitation counselor. In contrast to most mental institutions, The Club encourages members to express their feelings to staff in an open way. Disagreements tend to be aired and resolved. This practice seems to contribute to the generally high morale of personnel at The Club.

There is not a clear split at The Club between professional and paraprofessional staff members. Except for the psychiatrist, all personnel are considered habilitation counselors or habilitation supervisors. The Club's staff psychiatrist is involved in an unusually wide range of Club activities. Most psychosocial rehabilitation programs use a psychiatrist as a consultant who deals with psychiatric problems while the program maintains its focus on rehabilitation efforts. The Club has attempted to integrate these two activities more closely by involving the staff psychiatrist in much more of the program, and having her consult with habilitation workers about the psychiatric status of the members.

Evaluation

Little formal evaluation of the program or of the staff members is done. As with most of the centers visited during the research for this book, few resources tend to be allocated to formal evaluation procedures for staff members, or for the program. The Rutgers Mental Health Center evaluates its staff members annually. The Club uses the same evaluation form as the rest of the center. In general, habilitation workers are rated very well.

An interesting and unique feature of The Club evaluation is that Club members help in the gathering and writing of the monthly statistical reports which describe attendance, employment, and other relevant variables. While there is talk of doing so, to date there has been no formal evaluation of the program's impact. It has been considered impractical to undertake an evaluation because it is difficult to determine what constitutes a "satisfactory impact" on a client. While the ability to hold a job and support oneself are not synonymous with success, these outcomes are indicators of one's ability to function in society. They also are a saving to society because the individual does not need custodial care. Some impressive data are available. For example, Club members in transitional employment jobs earned over $10,000 during November 1976. Jobs within the mental health center and drivers for The Club yielded approximately another $2,000. Out of an active membership of 139 that month, two were rehospitalized. During that month, 67 members lived in SERV apartments and 40 members were involved in the education program. There is anecdotal evidence that the program has kept many clients out of the state hospital who would have had to return without The Club's support. The members' personal sense of satisfaction at having a job and living in an independent apartment is difficult to measure but seems to be very important.

Perhaps most impressive of all is the sense of self-worth and self-confidence that The Club instills in members who have a previous history of institutional dependency. There is a definite undercurrent of pride in their voices as members conduct tours of their Club and talk about their paying jobs and new apartments. The Club does not merely aim at keeping people out of the hospital, it tries to assist members to build social networks of friends and acquaintances, and to live as productive and independent a life as possible.

In Conclusion

The Club uses paraprofessional staff extensively in a wide variety of services designed to support clients in making a functional adjustment to living in the community. Services are much broader than those typically considered to be therapeutic, and include assistance in housing, transportation, work, and education. Carefully selected and trained paraprofessionals are ideal staff for such a program since traditional professional training is not an adequate preparation for this multifaceted approach.

Chapter 7

DRUG ABUSE SERVICES

INTRODUCTION

Description of the Service Area

Drug abuse programs have historically made extensive and successful use of paraprofessionals. They often are begun and run entirely by paraprofessionals, usually as independent organizational entities which are not directly connected with a community mental health center. When the need for a drug program is not already sufficiently met in the catchment area by a previously established organization, the community mental health center is responsible for providing these services.

To satisfy the National Institute of Mental Health requirements in this service area, a federally funded community mental health center must designate at least one staff member as administratively responsible for implementation of a drug program. This drug program should be coordinated with other appropriate service areas, such as outpatient, inpatient, emergency, and particularly with consultation and education. This latter connection should lead to planned preventive strategies in the community. Arrangements must be made to provide rapid evaluation and treatment by a psychiatrist or physician for medical and psychiatric complications resulting from drug abuse. In addition, the provision of detoxification services must be arranged.

Selection of the Site Visited

Selection of an appropriate site as a model for drug abuse treatment services started with requests for information and suggestions from all ten of the regional Health, Education, and Welfare offices, as well as from the National Institute of Drug Abuse. Projects in Chicago, Philadelphia, New York, Miami, and San Francisco were recommended. In addition, further searching turned up several projects in smaller cities.

One generalization to be made as a result of the telephone interviews is the emphasis most of these projects place on the treatment of heroin addicts by ex-addicts. All of the programs in the major cities were based on the therapeutic community treatment modality. Thus, the need to find a drug abuse program that deals with the ever-increasing population of nonaddictive (e.g., prescription) drug abusers became an important consideration.

None of the programs recommended were part of a community mental health center. This became another important selection criterion—could the program be useful as a model for a center's drug abuse services?

It was decided, after telephone interviews, as well as after the reading of a lengthy program description from a recent grant application, that Project Eden, located in Hayward, California, was the program that best satisfied our selection criteria.

Although Project Eden has a therapeutic community as one aspect of its program, the major emphasis is on the treatment of youthful poly-drug[1] abusers on an outpatient basis. The organization of the project is similar to many community mental health centers, providing a good example of service coordination, staff selection, training, education, supervision, and career mobility.

The project has an enormous degree of community support and involvement. It has been in operation for eight years and has evolved in response to community needs. Prevention and community education, including a well-established in-school program, are integral aspects of the project's services.

Project Eden is essentially a paraprofessional and volunteer organization. The executive director and all regular staff members, with two exceptions, are paraprofessionals. There are a number of professional persons who are regularly used on a consulting basis. They have had a long-term involvement with the project.

---

[1]Poly-drug is the present term used to describe the wide variety of chemical substances ingested by individuals without medical supervision. This term is usually not used to describe heroin addicts.

PROJECT EDEN: A CASE STUDY IN DRUG ABUSE SERVICES*

Prior to 1975, most community mental health centers did not provide drug abuse treatment services. Drug programs were usually begun by those outside the mental health establishment, funded by alternate sources, and staffed by nonprofessionals. Drug clients are often viewed as being "different" from clients with mental health problems and therefore they are segregated in their treatments. The staff members of drug treatment centers also tend to be different in background and life-style from other mental health personnel.

Project Eden is a drug program located about 10 miles south of Oakland in Hayward, California. The staff members, almost all of whom are paraprofessionals, provide a wide variety of direct and indirect services to a diversified clientele. Although Project Eden is an independent agency, it might serve as a model for a drug program in a more traditional community mental health center.

The catchment area consists of six Northern California suburban cities with a total population of 276,000. Youth make up 33% of the population, and 1970 figures indicate that 28% of persons aged 25–44 living in the area had not finished high school.

Project Eden provides services without restriction to all persons in the community who seek assistance for drug-related problems. The primary emphasis of Project Eden's services is aimed at the poly-drug users aged 15 to 24. In addition, emphasis is placed on services to Spanish-American drug abusers within this general category and hard drug users in the 24–35 age range.

Background

Project Eden was started at the end of the 1960s. The first wave of the drug abuse epidemic crested in the Hayward area in 1968. The incidence of drug use soared and the resulting overdose deaths caused widespread concern. Numerous members of the community met to consider strategies to cope with the newly emerging drug problem. School officials in particular desired an alternative to the expulsion of youth who were obvious users and sellers. The numbers involved made this traditional stopgap measure impractical.

The original planning group included a cross section of the community: the chief of police, probation officers, school administrators, a local physician, and concerned citizens. The labors of this group resulted in a community fund-raising drive that netted $25,000, and Project Eden was formed. The wide

*Contact: Project Eden, Inc.
         22738 Mission Blvd.
         Hayward, California   94541
         415/538-3818
         Attention: Lloyd Churgin, Executive Director

involvement of key community leaders from the outset is very probably a significant factor in the program's continued support.

Today the 27-member board of directors of Project Eden is composed of educators, physicians, mental health professionals, local officials, agency representatives, union representatives, attorneys, and other local citizens representing a broad, diversified base of interest and representation from the target community. The board is responsible for major policy formulation, fiscal monitoring, hiring of the executive director, and hiring review of management personnel.

Project Eden's initial operations consisted of a drop-in center and 24-hour telephone service, which included telephone counseling, drug information, and service referrals. The original program staff consisted of a director who was brought in from the East Coast, one other paid position, and volunteers. The volunteers were mostly middle-class youth with little formal education beyond high school. They began their efforts in response to the need as they saw it: "People were dying, man!" This core group developed a strong sense of family. There was a large commitment required in terms of time, energy, and emotion. Differences were worked out by a process called "grouping," wherein everyone met together and verbally, in what were described as highly charged and confrontive sessions, dealt with their feelings and, incidentally, program difficulties. The group was youth-oriented and interested in building a strong community base. All persons who wished to participate were required to be completely drug-free. This was often the only distinction between being a volunteer and being a client. The staff lived together. Volunteer staff members received help from those staff members already professionally trained. Until quite recently, there was little distinction in terms of service roles: "Everybody did everything."

The growth and evolution of program services has largely been in response to community needs. As a large number of heroin addicts started to "crash" at their center, Project Eden developed a structured residential treatment program. An emergency rescue service was started to deal with drug overdoses. Outpatient counseling was developed to assist individuals who were not necessarily in crisis, but who needed help to confront drug abuse problems. A comprehensive program of drug education and prevention supplemented the intervention services. To begin to deal with some of the reasons for the drug problem—no jobs and lack of job skills—Project Eden started an employment and training program. The school program grew out of an original request to help with recreational activities.

Project Eden is a community-based program that uses the resources of a paraprofessional and professional staff to attract and hold clients, the program responds quickly and effectively to the changing needs of individual clients as well as of the entire population, and maintains contact with this client population over a period of time so that these people may be successfully reintegrated into community life.

Of special significance in establishing rapport with this clientele is the existence of an open, informal, drug-free setting populated by paraprofessional staff members and volunteers from the local community who are about the same age as most of the clients. For many young drug users, Project Eden represents the first peer social setting where drug use is not reinforced or used as a criterion for belonging.

Project Eden is an interesting mix of values, goals, customs, and perceptions. This mix represents remnants from the early familial atmosphere as well as the results of growth and change through time. Although some people feel that Project Eden is now "nothing like it was," the emotional atmosphere is still strikingly open and honest. The total commitment to honesty has evolved so that staff members are encouraged to look at themselves, yet given permission not to until they are ready. Part of the reason for this change has been aptly described by the director: "If you spend 18 hours a week in a group emoting, the clients don't get the help."

Another change is Project Eden's attitude to the amount of time and energy spent by the staff working on the project. The original conditions were compared to a pressure cooker. It was a self-imposed pressure cooker required by the nature of the challenge. The staff had an almost missionary zeal and fervor to convert the "heathen drug takers" so the converts would forevermore lead a drug-free and productive life. At first there were few alternative methods available for drug treatment. There was also the need to keep a no-salary program together. But there were many casualties among staff members from this approach. The members often felt that they were doing much more than they were actually accomplishing. Since everyone was doing everything, it was difficult to evaluate the work. The people wasted energy defending ideological positions. Personnel would "burn out" and leave over minor issues, saying they had been used.

As the program evolved, small salaries became available and new people were hired. Today there is more emphasis on skilled staff or the potential of the staff member to develop skills based on training. Project Eden now uses more conventional, if less charismatic staff members. They are encouraged to be involved in interests away from and other than the project. Salaries are being upgraded to a level where "people don't have to starve, but they shouldn't get fat here either." The demand for a drug-free commitment has been recently modified. Deciding about marijuana usage is now considered each person's individual responsibility.

A particularly important change concerns job responsibilities. The staff members now specialize. At first each staff member did all of the different tasks. A person would work on switchboard, do some counseling, work in the schools, help with building maintenance. Everyone eventually agreed that this spread people too thin. So the one person/one job concept came into operation. Staff members concentrate in a particular area. However, there is a carryover from the past in that considerable flexibility still exists. If help is needed in a specific area, other staff members, including supervisors and the executive director, will lend a hand.

The community orientation is another important aspect of Project Eden. It is apparent in many facets of the program's operation. There is excellent rapport between staff members and the board of directors, which is composed of a cross section of the community. Relationships with other agencies in the community are actively sought and continuously cultivated. The crisis referral system benefits from this. The police department readily acknowledges the importance of Project Eden. When the police work with the rescue service, they normally do not make arrests. This "no bust" policy increases Project Eden's credibility on the streets. Project Eden approached the local school system cautiously, gradually establishing contact with all key personnel. This procedure ensured a good working relationship with teachers and administrators, minimizing unnecessary difficulties.

The project places a great emphasis on being in touch with life on the streets. It is from this sector of the community that the project arose. This is where the majority of the volunteers come from, and they are considered the "life blood" of the project. Programs have been developed, modified, and abandoned as the street scene has changed. The project encourages a drop-in atmosphere. Appointments are kept to a minimum. The building is open to anyone to come in and just "hang out." There are no demands. No one tries to proselytize the visitors. The staff members are just available, if help is requested. A TV, a stereo, several comfortable couches, and a pool table all contribute to this atmosphere. There are problems, usually associated with derelict alcoholics or others "crashing" for more than a day. These are deliberately dealt with in an easygoing fashion and are considered a necessary part of the cost of this type of program.

Often staff members will feel it is time to move on because they sense they have lost contact with the streets. A staff member aged 23, 24, or 25 already feels a generation removed from the 15-, 16-, and 17-year-olds. They may no longer be confident of their street savvy. It was recently suggested that perhaps workers should spend one day a week out in the community, hanging out, getting known, publicizing the program, and generally maintaining contact with the changing scene. On the other hand, the director feels that the job should not be a sinecure and that personnel change should be a normal pattern.

Project Eden has been strongly defined as a *drug* program. While this is a positive value as far as funding is concerned, it is not always the best image to attract clientele. One reason is the impression of youth that "drugs equal heroin." Soft-drug users do not want to become identified with or involved in a heroin program. Another negative aspect of a drug program is that a young person may deny drug use as a problem in itself. They don't like to go where they feel they will be labeled as drug problems.

Project Eden would like to deemphasize its drug services aspect and be identified more as a youth services program. They feel that this would give them a better street image. They also feel it would be closer to what they really do, closer to what really needs to be done in the community. Drug counselors are well aware that drug use is only the most easily identifiable problem and often covers a variety of other specific life-style problems. Besides, why should alienated and unemployed youth have to become drug abusers in order to receive guidance and help with their problems?

Program Organization and Services

Project Eden provides residential and outpatient services as well as preventive and community education programs. The residential services consist of a halfway house, a therapeutic community, and a family store. These programs are housed in separate facilities apart from the outpatient/administrative building. There are 16 employees who staff the residential program, all paraprofessionals. The outpatient services are divided into four components: crisis/switchboard, counseling, school youth intervention, and employment/training. Twenty staff members are employed in the outpatient services. All are paraprofessionals except the director, who has a master's degree in counseling, and the employment coordinator, who is a social worker. Psychiatric and medical consultation is provided as needed by a social worker and a medical doctor who have been involved for a long time with the program. The drug education program is coordinated by a single paraprofessional. Program administration consists of the executive director (a paraprofessional who has been with the program since its first year), his administrative assistant, an office manager, and a bookkeeper. There is also a maintenance coordinator who recently has been in charge of extensive interior building renovation. (Outpatient services make use of 35 volunteers, mostly community youth, who are primarily involved in the crisis/switchboard component.)

Project Eden operates a switchboard for crisis calls, phone counseling, drug information, and referrals. The switchboard was the original program service, run by volunteers in an abandoned school biology building. It has operated continuously, 24 hours a day, seven days a week since May 1970. The switchboard is staffed by a paid paraprofessional supervisor, who has full responsibility, and by volunteers.

In addition to switchboard workers, at least two trained crisis teams are on duty around the clock and the project maintains a vehicle which is used solely to respond to emergency calls in the community. A formal arrangement is maintained whereby an ambulance may be dispatched to respond to potentially life-threatening situations.

The two or three person crisis team may be made up entirely of volunteers. At least one volunteer is designated as a "first person." This person has had considerable crisis experience (going out on crisis calls as a "second person" with assisting responsibilities, or a "third person" with minimal responsibilities besides observation); has been trained in crisis techniques such as cardiopulmonary resuscitation, first aid, street drug pharmacology, etc.; has undergone a 13-week volunteer training group; has been evaluated by the switchboard supervisors and determined to be a responsible individual; and commands the respect of the other volunteers. The "first person" will phone the switchboard after the initial contact is made and immediate first aid is administered. The decision to send an ambulance and/or to hospitalize is up to the supervisor and in general the supervisor is considered the final authority.

Information and referrals are available to both telephone inquirers and drop-in clients. Many of the callers are isolated people who use the switchboard to ventilate or rap with staff. This is in addition to a large number of persons seeking information and referrals regarding drug abuse and related problems.

Many drop-in clients are in a state of crisis when they arrive at the project. They are often brought in by friends or relations who have heard of Project Eden and have nowhere else to turn. A typical case at present is a client who has taken too much PCP (phenylcyclidine)—an animal tranquilizer.

Project Eden has had to define for itself the concept and purpose of counseling in order to decide on criteria for accepting clients. The most effective counseling approach found for meeting the needs of the target population is the paraprofessional, peer counseling model that essentially addresses the social and interpersonal aspects of drug abuse and its underlying and related problems.

Counselors are therefore trained to deal with problems of social development that can most accurately be described as counseling for personalities that are relatively intact and healthy. This program is not designed or equipped to treat deep-seated psychopathology that requires professional psychotherapy. Typically, individuals with extensive psychiatric treatment histories or those who present non-drug-related intrapsychic disturbances would be appropriate referrals for professional treatment. Often the program's clinical consultant is called in for evaluation and recommendation for referral on these cases.

Individual and group problem-solving focuses on those individuals seeking resolution of specific situational, personal, and/or emotional difficulties. Initial contact is usually made during a period of crisis and first sessions are often devoted to defining and understanding underlying causes and problems. Once the terms and focus of the counseling relationship are established, the duration is most often dictated by the needs of the client. Also, significant people in the client's life, such as parents and friends, may be involved by the counselor and client when it is appropriate.

Family counseling is usually initiated due to the drug use of an immediate family member. In situations where the drug-using family member is seeing a counselor, the family counseling becomes an adjunct or takes place concurrently with the individual's counseling sessions. If the drug-using family member is not seeking counseling assistance, the family counseling process becomes somewhat more supportive and oriented towards the development of decision-making tools for non-drug-using family members who are being affected by the situation.

Individuals who clearly do not desire structured counseling are usually encouraged to become involved in less structured individual or group rap sessions. These rap sessions in Project Eden are primarily focused on developing trusting relationships and socialization skills rather than dealing with specific problem areas. Often clients, at first reluctant to become involved in structured counseling, eventually seek it out after developing some rapport and trust through open rap sessions. Rap sessions may occur spontaneously throughout the day between counseling staff and clients, and an open drop-in rap session is scheduled weekly in the evening for anyone who wishes to attend.

Project Eden has been involved since its inception with the school system. School administrative personnel shared responsibility for the original organization effort. This was in response to the increasingly obvious drug-related problems evidenced in the behavior of students.

Involvement in a school system by a social service organization always requires careful planning and sensitivity. The project staff increased their chances of successful involvement in a number of ways. They worked closely with school district administrators in setting up the outreach program. They asked for input from the school principals in the development of the program. The principals interviewed and approved each of the paraprofessionals who worked in their schools. Funding for the program came out of existing Project Eden money, and thus there was no cost to the schools. Lines of communication between project and schools were clearly established. In the event of any problem, each principal knew whom to call, and was assured of immediate response and assistance. Finally, rather than trying to present the program design to the schools, the staff requested six months for the paraprofessionals to reconnoiter their school and determine its particular needs and resources.

There are at present (as of January 1, 1977) eight outreach counselors in four high schools, two of which are continuation schools. It is the hope of the outreach team that by establishing themselves as a positive, useful influence in the high schools, they will be able to eventually work in the junior high schools and elementary schools where early-age prevention via education can become more meaningful.

The personal qualities and attitudes of the outreach counselor are the most important measure in regards to success of this type of program. Counselors must be mature individuals capable of working with administration, regular school counselors, and teachers, as well as with the school youth population. Many outreach counselors have grown up in the area and have attended the specific school in which they work so that they are familiar with the situation. However, with this background they must keep aware of their possible prejudices towards teachers, principals, and other personnel and must determine if they are capable of working in a somewhat delicate middle ground position. The outreach counselors also have to deal with the prejudices of the teachers and principals and often have had to spend time proving themselves.

Outreach counselors do a number of different tasks depending upon the school. In some schools they work as tutors. This gives them an initial contact with students, who learn to talk to them and to trust them. The knowledge that counselors are a resource for job training (see employment program description) often causes students to seek them out. In a continuation high school, the counselor supervises a drop-in room that is solely used for the program. This is a place for students to hang out, an alternative to outright truancy. As much as possible, this room is not identified as for drug users. No formal identification of this type is used. Counseling, job training, and tutoring, for example, are offered to anyone who needs and requests such help. A drug user identification, as well as identification along ethnic or school clique lines, can be a problem in trying to operate a program with broad appeal.

The school counselors do counseling similar to that at the outpatient center. They deal with employment, health, family crises, school problems, drug problems—almost anything that comes their way. They must recognize their limitations and make use of referrals when necessary. Project Eden workers have found that establishing trust and a good reputation are important keys to success.

Project Eden works in cooperation with the county Youth Employment Training Program. An experienced social worker from this program has an office at Project Eden's center. Project Eden uses its counseling services in conjunction with job training, because former drug users often have trouble getting jobs—or even job training. A problem related to job training is that county government guidelines require the identification of those accepted into the program as "poly-drug users." Needless to say, this label is a source of discomfort to trainees. They are concerned with future negative implications if their previous history becomes known.

The employment coordinator relies on the outreach counselors, particularly in the continuation high schools, for job training applicants. She reports being flooded with requests, and has to carefully interview those admitted into the program. Governmental regulations, due to funding sources, also require careful initial screening to fill various quotas.

The employment coordinator has worked hard on relationships with many local industries. Her knowledge of the personalities and expertise of supervisors responsible for training in these industries aids in successful placement. Training also takes place in classroom settings such as the local business college. Trainees are assisted in obtaining high school diplomas through the graduate equivalency test (General Educational Development or GED).

The Project has one full-time paraprofessional staff member responsible for a drug education program. This individual is responsible for a broad range of community education activities including: coordination of the Community

Speakers Bureau; publishing the *Plain Rapper,* the Project newsletter; liaison with four local parent-teacher association councils; liaison with the business community and service organizations; liaison with area church groups; liaison with students, teachers, and administrators in three local school districts; development of printed and visual drug education materials; and contact with San Francisco Bay area print and electronic media.

The primary focus of the drug education program is threefold: first, to provide accurate information regarding drug abuse to the local community; second, to publicize the availability of services offered by Project Eden; and third, to maintain active contact with various segments of the community to assure continual feedback regarding the appropriateness and responsiveness of project services to the changing local drug scene.

It is strongly felt that much of the heavy use of project services, and a good deal of the community support and involvement in the project, may be attributed to the efforts and accomplishments of this service component.

To provide treatment services for drug addicts, Project Eden established a halfway house and also a therapeutic community. The majority of successful clients using these establishments are court referrals. It is still felt, though, that clients who voluntarily commit themselves to the highly structured and disciplined environments have a good chance of moving through the programs.

Use of Paraprofessionals

There are three types of people who are employed at Project Eden: the old timer, the newcomer, and the old timer newly arrived.

The Old Timers.   These are the staff members who have been around the program practically since its beginning. Before coming to the program, most of these people were involved in drugs or some other form of behavior that might be considered nonproductive and self-damaging. Five years with the program is a common length of service with the project. These staff members are able to "remember it when." They recall that Synanon was the initial model for Project Eden and remember this initial phase as a time when people were close, emotional, trusted each other, and were able to scream when they felt that the trust was broken.

After the length of time they have been in the program, they express feelings of being tired—but not burned out. These are the staff members with stamina. Those who have burned out left long ago. Although they are very knowledgeable in terms of their tasks, the old timers speak openly of being away from the streets for a long time. At age 23, for example, one old-time counselor is able to speak at length about three generations of drug users that have been tripping out since the heyday of the Haight-Ashbury scene in San Francisco.

Old timers are inevitably full of personal plans. They have used Project Eden as a safe place to grow. Now they are ready to leave. The sense of continuing to help others is deeply ingrained. One counselor is going to try real estate. She will sell homes to "gay," "hip," and interracial couples—anyone she feels is mistreated by the majority of present realtors.

The Newcomer.   Many paraprofessional workers in community mental health centers are recruited today from the ranks of the unemployed or underemployed college-educated population. These people usually do not start with the program as volunteers. They may have worked previously in a similar program as part of a field placement or internship. They tend to be young, bright, and interested in "doing something meaningful with their lives" —this latter phrase perhaps also best describes everyone who has worked at Project Eden. The newcomers see Eden as a challenge and feel good about the comparison of the project with more formal organizations where they have previously been employed. In contrast to other bureaucracies—offices or schools—Project Eden seems like the "Garden of Eden." "The director just comes in and drinks coffee with us," says one staffer. To the newcomer the openness of the program staff is astonishing.

These staff members tend to work extra hours. They try their skill at creating new projects. They feel they have the freedom and the support to be innovative.

The Old Timer Newly Arrived.   At some point in the evolution of Project Eden, the executive director felt that he needed to hire personnel skilled enough to handle middle management positions. The resource for this type of recruitment is the counselor who has been through the ropes with other alternative programs. This type of person is a changer and a doer. There is a sense of commitment to a life-style that continually tries to improve things. This person will shake things up and run things right. Their orientation is to work constructively and cooperatively towards a resolution of problems. Meaningful program changes occur due to these staff members. They have experience, energy, skill, and ambition.

Volunteers.   A mainstay of Project Eden's ability to deliver services over the years has been its heavy reliance on trained volunteer workers. Street credibility is greatly enhanced by training young people from the community to work on their own turf with people who they often know who are having problems with drugs. Trained, dedicated volunteers, familiar with program operations, are an invaluable resource group from which to hire staff. A majority of the current project staff started with the program as volunteers. Additionally, the volunteer program provides an opportunity for young people to contribute to dealing with community problems and, at the same time, to continue their own personal growth.

Affirmative Action.   In an effort to gain entrance into the Latin neighborhoods, Project Eden offered assistance to help local Chicano groups with information, training, and technical assistance. They discovered many separate organizations involved in a great deal of in-fighting. One group asked Project Eden to help by running off gun manuals on their photocopying machine. The staff felt it was impossible to work with these disparate groups. Instead, Project Eden is diversifying its own staff to include more Chicanos and other minorities. In this way they will have the appropriate personnel who can respond to the needs of the minority communities.

A major affirmative action program has been accepted by the board of directors. Ethnic hiring quotas have been set representing the population percentages of the area, and are being filled at each level of the project, from the board of directors to the volunteers.

Training

Training is a primary responsibility for the clinical consultant. He is a psychiatric social worker who has been working with Project Eden almost from the start of the program. Training sessions are held once a week. The trainer prepares a manual for each series of sessions. The manual outlines the purpose and goals of the session. It contains space for the trainees to write in personal goals. There is a section for the trainee to keep a personal journal.

Many subjects are covered in training. Counseling techniques and clinical issues are discussed. Case summaries are reviewed and analyzed. Role playing and psychodrama are used to help counselors keep aware of how they appear to others.

When enough new volunteers have been accepted into the program, the trainer runs a volunteers group with the assistance of two counselors. He spends an hour before and an hour after the group session with the counselors, discussing what has occurred. The group itself is organized to discuss the issues involved in being a volunteer, to provide training in techniques, to provide a place to express feelings, to provide a feeling of togetherness with other volunteers, to meet the project staff, and to provide a place for evaluation by counselors and trainers of volunteers. At the end of 8 to 12 sessions there are 12 to 20 trained volunteers as well as two counselors who have gained valuable experience.

The crisis switchboard supervisors all receive training as volunteers. Besides the formal training, they learn on the job. Training by doing is an important aspect of Project Eden. Workers are carefully supervised, however, to protect clients against inexperienced personnel. Volunteers who work on the switchboard taking calls and making referrals are supervised until it is felt that they have enough experience to make responsible decisions. Crisis teams have a "first person," "second person," "third person" hierarchy. To move from observer status to the leader of a crisis team requires that the person demonstrate responsibility, so that the switchboard supervisor, as well as the other volunteers, trusts that person's ability to make decisions and act in life and death situations.

Supervision

The staff members in each component of Project Eden meet once a week with their coordinator. The coordinators then prepare reports for a weekly meeting with the executive director.

The atmosphere at the center is open and flexible, providing the program staff members opportunity for continual and on-going problem-solving. The outpatient director reports that sometimes he feels as though he spends up to three quarters of his time working with staff members on their interpersonal problems. His availability and warmth encourage the staff members to talk to him. Thus, he is able to keep track of what is going on and can also institute change by suggesting an approach or ideas to staff members.

The staff members in the different components make an effort to get together. When time permits, they have group discussions about issues of joint concern. These meetings can create an atmosphere of questioning that fights complacency.

Mobility

The components provide for an in-program mobility that is unrelated to salary increases. The majority of the staff came into Project Eden as volunteers. They came for philosophical and personal reasons: to do something meaningful with their lives and to help others. As a staff member becomes more adept at crisis work and gains more knowledge of the program, there is the move from "third person" to "first person" status. "First person" volunteers recognize the responsibility of their position. They are proud of their work; they find it exciting and challenging.

"First person" volunteers are hired to be switchboard supervisors. They are already familiar with the job, but the salary and decision making responsibility provide the step up.

Switchboard supervisors can either remain with their component and advance to the position of coordinator, or may move on to the counseling component. Outpatient counselors in turn can work as outreach counselors in the school. This procedure gives people program skills in a wide variety of areas. They are thus equipped to work in positions of responsibility elsewhere, or use their knowledge if they return to school.

Education

Many paraprofessionals who work in the program have been previously "turned off" by school. Their experiences with the formal educational system were usually negative. Through Project Eden they have gained many of the skills and the positive self-image that their formal schooling did not provide. For example, there is peer pressure to write up case work notes so that others are able to read and understand them; working on a budget brings a need for mathematics; relating to other ethnic groups requires a foreign language; public speaking requires a good command of English; an understanding of the changing drug culture requires sociological sophistication; counselors and others who work with people in crisis are gaining knowledge of the field of psychology. This type of education is really at the core of the appeal of Project Eden to its staff. They value highly what they have learned. More than salary or sinecure, the staff members report that the challenge of learning, the need to learn in order to help others, continues to keep interest and morale at a high level.

It is the stated policy of Project Eden to give paid time off to its staff personnel in order to further their education. More than that, academic learning is encouraged. It is felt that education from outside the program makes staff better able to serve their clients.

The director feels that his staff would benefit more from a broad general education such as that available from a junior college, rather than from training that is limited to the skills necessary to be a drug counselor. The intensive experience they receive in the drug field through the project would be better supplemented with a general education. A general education would improve job performance in such areas as writing, conceptualizing, communicating, and planning. It would also assist the workers in the area of job mobility. The director feels that his staff is qualified to work in a variety of human service areas, not just drug treatment.

One staff member became involved in a specialized type of training program. He was to receive college credit for his six years experience working in the drug program. Unfortunately, the massive amount of paperwork required to document his experience was just too overwhelming. He now plans to attend junior college to, in part, "work on my writing skills."

Credentialing.   At present the executive director is working on the problem of formally acknowledging the level of skills that the paraprofessionals have gained from their experiences. He is on a statewide committee that is exploring various possibilities and developing guidelines. Program accreditation is one possibility. However, personnel at Project Eden fear that accreditation would freeze a program into a particular organizational design, and that the best design is as yet unknown. Credentialing gives status to paraprofessionals and provides security. It also limits the functions they may perform and can close off the field to others. The executive director hopes to develop, with local colleges, an A.A. degree model that demands a level of competency, but works against specialization by making those credentialed eligible to work in a wide variety of human service areas.

Status

The paraprofessional and professional staff at Project Eden do not seem to have problems around the issue of status. Paraprofessionals like and admire the two full-time staff members with advanced degrees—the social worker who coordinates the employment program, and the director of outpatient services. The clinical consultant, a psychiatric social worker, and the medical consultant have all been with the project since its inception and they are also well respected.

Staff members complain of trouble in dealing with psychiatrists and psychologists in other agencies. They all report the experience of being talked down to and not being taken seriously. This attitude angers them but they are quick to state that they also have good relationships with outside professionals. Some professionals call and ask for advice and help when their patients have drug-related problems. Some refer clients to the program.

When Project Eden began, only the executive director received a salary. Until recently the staff salaries continued to reflect this initial orientation by providing scarcely enough money for the workers to live on. Part of this was due to the philosophy that Eden was something to commit your life to, and that, therefore, money was not necessary. Gradually, as funds have become available, the executive director is trying to upgrade salaries so that they are comparable to similar programs in the San Francisco Bay Area.

Since the project is funded from several local, state, and federal sources, personnel in different components and even within the components receive different salaries. That this is not more of an issue strongly indicates that staff members are involved in Eden for other than monetary reasons.

Evaluation

Project Eden constantly evaluates the relevancy and effectiveness of its drug intervention services. They see evaluation as an important tool in providing flexible services that are responsive to the changing needs and conditions of the local drug scene. The evaluation of services takes place in three separate areas:

1. A client feedback form has been designed which allows clients to record anonymous comments, suggestions, and criticisms of project services. Client feedback is also solicited informally in conversations with clients and drop-ins, and the results of this feedback are often discussed at staff meetings.
2. Each component meets on a weekly basis to share perceptions and problem solving difficulties within the component.
3. There is an informal system to solicit feedback and suggestions from the general public regarding project services. Complaints that are received by

telephone are recorded. Feedback is solicited by the Speakers Bureau when talks are given to community groups.

In Conclusion

Project Eden represents an example of varied groups of people working together to attempt to deal effectively with serious community problems. The combination of the support and interest of a broad-based citizens' board, the energy and talents of volunteer and paid paraprofessional staff members, and the knowledge and experience of mental health professionals should serve as a model for similar efforts.

Chapter 8

EMERGENCY SERVICES

INTRODUCTION

Description of the Service Area

A community mental health center must provide immediate evaluation and mental health care for persons in crisis on a 24-hour, seven-day-a-week basis. This emergency service must include both face-to-face crisis intervention, as well as a "hotline" telephone service. Face-to-face services may be provided at one central emergency room or walk-in clinic, or, for those centers serving large geographical areas, several facilities might be necessary. In addition, a mobile crisis team should be available to handle mental health emergencies that arise in the community. A 24-hour crisis telephone service should be established with one central service and both should have a single telephone number. This is to decrease the possibility of losing clients who may become frustrated trying to reach the correct person in order to receive help. Mental health personnel should be available immediately to assist persons in crisis over the telephone.

All components of the emergency service should be coordinated into a unified program which, in turn, should be coordinated with other appropriate service elements, that is, outside agencies. It is important that, as their needs dictate, patients receiving emergency care can be transferred readily to other services at the center.

Selection of the Site Visited

The Southwest Denver Community Mental Health Services Center was chosen as the site to visit in the emergency services delivery area. The Southwest Denver Center has used paraprofessional staff members in a comprehensive fashion since its inception. The tasks within the center are performed by those persons with the necessary, desired skills. The selection of the majority of program staff members is based not upon academic credentials, but on individual competency in requisite skills.

The center's emergency program philosophy is based upon the extensive use of crisis therapy performed in the social setting in which the problem is found. The therapy, therapist, and setting in which the therapy occurs are tailored to each client's needs. Much therapy takes place in the client's home.

There is a group of families used by the center who provide an alternative, healthy environment for clients in crisis when circumstances require that they be removed from their usual environment. The integration of these alternative family homes for inpatient services with emergency and outpatient services has reduced the mental hospital referrals from the catchment area to less than one bed at any one time per 100,000 population.

In addition, the emergency program meets the standards set by National Institute of Mental Health guidelines and was recommended highly by the Department of Health, Education, and Welfare deputy director of Region VIII and by Judy Turner of the Mental Health Services Support branch, NIMH, Washington, D.C.

SOUTHWEST DENVER COMMUNITY MENTAL HEALTH SERVICES, INC.: A CASE STUDY IN EMERGENCY SERVICES*

Comprehensive mental health services are provided for the 109,000 (1976 census) citizens in the southwest Denver area by a unique service delivery system known as Southwest Denver Community Mental Health Services, Inc. (SWDCMHS). The essential components of the program include the use of community homes as alternatives to inpatient hospitalization; home, or "social system" based outpatient therapy; outreach crisis intervention; and the widespread use of paraprofessional staff members. The center believes in citizen

*Contact: Southwest Denver Community Mental Health Services, Inc.
　　　　 1611 South Federal
　　　　 Denver, Colorado   80219
　　　　 303/922-7811
　　　　 Attention: Paul Polak, Center Director
　　　　　　　　　 Alice Jones, Program Director

participation and community control of its programs, and in the elimination of formal staff offices; it focuses on working with the client in the clients' real-life setting as much as possible. This chapter describes the provision of emergency services, as well as the use of the inpatient alternative homes program.

The intake/crisis program (emergency services) operates on a 24-hour basis making use of all the adult psychiatry services staff members to respond to crisis calls from the community. The adult psychiatry service is staffed by one psychologist, three social workers, seven registered nurses, and 14 paraprofessional staff members. A paraprofessional staff member, Alice Jones, is in charge of the intake/crisis program formally known as Entry and Intervention. Her duties include: managing a group that supervises clinicians, including professional staff members; administering the intake/crisis procedure; monitoring the caseloads of all the clinicians; acting as a "troubleshooter" for the difficult cases; and carrying a one-third time caseload.

The program provides mental health services to clients and to their families, with special attention paid to the social systems in which they function. The integration of services and follow-up is maximized by having the staff member who handles the intake/crisis call assume the client onto his/her ongoing caseload. The staff member is then responsible for developing a treatment plan and coordinating future services. When necessary, the staff member has available the use of one of six homes in the community. These serve as a temporary change of scene for a person in crisis without subjecting that person to the additional trauma of hospital admission.

Background

Before hiring its first staff member in 1966—the center director, Paul Polak, M.D.—citizens of southwest Denver engaged in an active three-year planning process. The present philosophy toward mental health services, which provides immediate, responsive service as close as possible to the home of the client, is in accord with the ideas evolved by the governing citizens board during the three-year planning process.

The philosophy of the center is a product of Dr. Polak's experiences and beliefs, the ideas of the community as represented by the board of directors, and an outgrowth of various plans, attempted with varying degrees of success, by the center staff members.

Dr. Polak's experience as director of research at nearby Fort Logan Mental Hospital in Denver gave him the opportunity to view, firsthand, some of the paradoxes of inpatient mental health treatment. These included the discrepancy between staff treatment goals for patients and the patients' goals for themselves; the identification of the patient as sick when the problem could be viewed as involving the entire immediate social system (for example, the individual's family or place of work); the stress the patient had to undergo when admitted into the hospital, and how this further exacerbated the problem (called the "crisis of admission"); and the serious loss of relevant information when an emergency client is interviewed away from the scene of the crisis. Dr. Polak's questioning of established psychiatric practices continued during his two-year stay at Dingleton Hospital in Scotland, where he worked with Maxwell Jones, a pioneer in the concept of therapeutic communities.

Upon his return from Scotland, Dr. Polak became the head of the Crisis Division at Fort Logan. He began to train a crisis team consisting of nurses and paraprofessional workers to handle mental health emergencies in the community setting where they occurred.

Many of the members of this team eventually became the staff members at SWDCMHS. At present, nine of these "old-timers" are on the staff. In particular, Alice Jones, who had many years of experience working in hospital settings, was hired by Dr. Polak to manage the intake/crisis program.

The concept of citizen participation and community control has always been important. The citizens board is not just an advisory group—it actually governs. It can hire and fire the director, set overall policy, and actively monitor ongoing programs. All 15 board members live in southwest Denver, eight representing specific neighborhoods and seven elected at large. Anyone who lives or works in southwest Denver may register to vote in board elections, and center clients are encouraged both to vote and to run for election to the board. Volunteers play a major role in all phases of the center's operation. Volunteer hours total over 1,000 per month, much of the time being directly involved in clinical work with clients. Clients are encouraged to become volunteers after their treatment and, in some instances, as part of their treatment.

The board of directors said in their initial statement: "We believe that the best place to treat the individual is within his own environment." The major treatment emphasis is on home visits. This is encouraged by the total lack of private offices for anyone but the administrative personnel. Experience taught that no matter what philosophy is stated, mental health workers, once ensconced in private offices, become highly territorial and rarely venture forth into the community. All clinical staff offices were eliminated, with space made available only for telephone and paper work.

Since the majority of individuals or families who become clients at mental health facilities do so in a state of crisis, a policy was formulated to provide immediate crisis services at the point of entry into treatment for all clients. Thus, most requests for services are evaluated within 24 hours, and the staff member handling the crisis is usually the coordinator for all subsequent treatment activities.

The philosophy of the intake/crisis program is based on previous theoretical research indicating that the "social systems" within which the client operates (such as the family, home environment, and working conditions), and the conflicts or difficulties in these situations, are often more potent determinants of the requests for mental health services than the intrapsychic problems of the individual identified as the patient. As a result, all the clinical workers stress including in the treatment program the relevant people around the client seeking help. The initial crisis-oriented evaluation procedure usually occurs in the setting of the social system involved.

The SWDCMHS makes use of all the available resources of the community to deal with the problems of persons in the community. They rely very little on the techniques of traditional psychiatry. The use of volunteers not only helps to cut costs, but also increases the self-esteem of those people who contribute their services.

SWDCMHS has 57 professional and paraprofessional staff, administrative, and clerical positions with an annual budget of approximately $860,000. There are 22 professional staff members who work with 20 paraprofessional staff workers. Top-level administration is the domain of either Ph.Ds or M.Ds. Separate programs are run by social workers or paraprofessionals who are titled "mangers." Programs are staffed by registered nurses, masters-level personnel, and paraprofessionals. Program staff members are almost entirely called "clinicians" and paid varying salaries based on experience, expertise, level of education, and the length of time with the program. The pay for clinicians who have completed training ranges from $10,600 to $13,000 with an average of $11,400. It is interesting that masters-level people are found at the high and low end of the pay scale with the paraprofessionals spaced between.

Since the staff clinicians are generalists working in all service delivery areas, on any one day a paraprofessional might be called upon to lead an activity program for severely regressed schizophrenics in a nursing home; visit a school to coordinate a treatment program for a preadolescent with the parents, school social worker, and teacher; make a home visit to meet with a family experiencing difficulties with an elderly parent showing signs of senility; hold an individual session with a client on probation for burglary and drug abuse; counsel a married couple; and visit a hospital emergency room to evaluate a client with slashed wrists.

As is apparent, being a community-oriented mental health clinician implies working with a broad spectrum of clients in all the settings they are located in, and being able to evaluate and devise a treatment program for each one of them. Given the tremendous variety of cases encountered and the equally diverse needs of clients, no single treatment, modality, or program is sufficient. The paraprofessionals need to draw upon their own creativity to devise a program relevant to the clients needs.

Program Organization and Services

Entry and Intervention, a division of Adult Psychiatry Services, provides intake evaluation and emergency services 24 hours a day, seven days a week. Accessibility to all treatment modalities of the center is provided through this entry system. A face-to-face evaluation is done by staff members who respond immediately to most crisis situations. Routine requests for treatment are evaluated within 24 hours, or at the convenience of the client. Clients are seen in their natural settings in a majority of cases (65% as of July 1976).

Statements from the staff reflect these basic goals: "We like to get them while they are hot!" "If you let it [the crisis] cool down, it refreezes and your effect can be greatly diminished." "The next crisis can be much worse because people didn't learn anything from the last one."

When a patient exhibits suicidal, homicidal, or psychotic behavior, it sometimes becomes necessary to remove him temporarily from his immediate social system. It is at this point that Southwest Denver Community Mental Health Services makes use of alternative families in lieu of hospital admission. This community alternative is seen as a backup for a strong crisis intervention approach in the patient's social environment. Traditional hospitalization is viewed only as the final resource to a community alternative system for intensive treatment. There were only 134 inpatient days during the last year.

Regardless of the modality to which the case is assigned, the clinician who has the first contact with the client remains the primary therapist. The client remains with the therapist until the case is closed. If clients call the center even after their cases are closed, they are referred back to their original therapists. This procedure insures a continuity of treatment to the client.

Procedure.   When a call comes in, a clinician interviews the person to determine the urgency of the situation. Clinicians use the basic classifications outlined below to assign priorities.

First priority is given to a "drop everything and go" crisis. These cases include any situation in which someone's life is in danger (an attempted homicide, suicide, or threats of violence). If weapons such as firearms are involved, the police are called and apprised of the situation before the clinician responds. Cases of a severe psychotic episode, referral calls from Denver General Hospital, and occurrences in public places complete the first category of crises.

Less urgent but still critical situations are considered to be nonimmediate emergencies, and are handled as quickly as possible, generally within 24 hours. The primary method of response is for the clinician to go to the home of the client to do a face-to-face evaluation. Following this visit the clinician can choose to do crisis therapy immediately, arrange for a later appointment (thus beginning an outpatient relationship), or refer the client to a crisis therapy group. The crisis therapy group meets two evenings a week for group therapy and gives persons in crisis the chance to meet and to interact with others in a similar situation. An alternative to treating a nonimmediate crisis in the home is to arrange for the client to come to the clinic as soon as possible to be evaluated and to begin a treatment program there.

In noncrisis situations, clients are seen at their convenience, but not necessarily within 24 hours. If it is determined that immediate therapy is not needed, there are several arrangements which are possible.

An appointment can be made with the client for a later date either in the client's social setting or in the clinic. Alternatively, an appointment can be scheduled for a medical evaluation to prescribe, increase, or decrease medication. Sometimes it is appropriate to refer the person to a crisis therapy group. Some calls can be answered by referral to another social service agency; occasionally, for example, a welfare social worker is needed to help solve a specific problem. In certain situations the person is given advice over the phone and no face-to-face contact is necessary.

In responding to a call and going to the environment in which the crisis is occurring, the clinician must first decide whether it is appropriate to be accompanied by a helper. There is a list of persons, primarily trained volunteers, available for assistance. As one clinician said, "It is sometimes a good idea to have a big guy with you." When asked how they deal with the anxiety of doing a crisis evaluation in a nonclinical setting, the clinicians mostly felt that "you don't, but you get used to it; and you can *always* count on backup."

When the clinicians respond to a major emergency, two questions very often need to be answered: Should the person be removed from the home? and Does the person need medication? It is the philosophy of the center to use medication and remove the person from the social setting only when absolutely necessary. If possible, the clinician will try to "talk him down." The clinicians try to see if the immediate crisis is indicative of a more general problem. At this point, ongoing outpatient therapy usually begins with the client who remains in the home.

If medication seems to be required, the clinician may, after consultation, arrange to bring the client to the center for a medical evaluation and have the doctor prescribe medication. If it is not appropriate to bring the client to the center, the clinic psychiatrist will do an evaluation in the home. Most medical evaluations are done in the center.

In the case of acute psychotic episodes, the doctor from the center will begin rapid tranquilization with a special constant observation team composed of a psychiatric nurse, clinicians, and specially trained volunteers who will observe the client constantly during the first day or two of treatment. The clinician and nurse are not always there but will check with the volunteer team every two to four hours. This rapid tranquilization procedure will often be done in the home or in an alternative home as opposed to being done in the hospital.

The client's family or friends also may be used as a resource throughout the rapid tranquilization procedure. In one instance, a husband stayed with his wife during most of her rapid tranquilization. Within three days her psychotic state/episode was essentially arrested; she then stayed with an alternative family until she was able to return to her own home. She later said she had felt better knowing her husband was nearby during the period of rapid tranquilization.

Alternative Homes.   Only occasionally does the Southwest Denver staff feel it is necessary to remove clients from their homes. Most often this occurs because there is no one to help the client in the home, the people in the home need respite, or the client requires medical attention. In most of these cases, clients are referred to alternative homes. Only a small minority of clients who would clearly be dangerous to the alternative family sponsors or who have a medical or physical problem requiring hospitalization are referred to the Fort Logan Mental Hospital.

When clients are removed from their own residence they are usually taken to one of the homes used by the Southwest Denver center as an alternative to inpatient hospitalization. This program began operating in February 1972. It is a system made up of families who take one or two psychiatric patients needing intensive treatment into their homes.

The homes are located close to the center's facilities and to the client's own neighborhood; each home setting provides a warm, consistent family structure for a maximum of two clients. Each client has a private room and is treated as a guest. The center pays the family $250 per month for making their homes available. This money is paid whether or not the home is needed for a client. An additional $7 is earned for each day two clients are in the home.

The homes are just that—homes. It is the intention that the alternative be a normal home environment, not a decentralized "mini" ward. According to the center's manager of inpatient alternative homes, clients going into the alternative homes view themselves as guests and generally behave like guests. This would contrast with the usual behavior of patients hospitalized for psychiatric disorders. The families (called home sponsors) are instructed to act not like therapists or hospital attendants but to be themselves, a family. To quote the head of inpatient alternatives, "We don't want to train these people to be 'professional' paraprofessionals. We want them to keep their 'people' skills. This is the key and the reason relationships are established which often last long after the client leaves."

The home sponsors do not receive any special training in therapeutic techniques. However, there are certain things they are taught by the coordinators and clinicians, such as the ability to recognize reactions to medication, precautions to use in the case of suicidal problems (removing razors), and procedures for emergencies (whom to call). Clinicians stress to the home sponsors that they should not view themselves as therapists. It is emphasized that the responsibility for the client rests ultimately with the clinician who must make all clinical decisions.

In addition to the general instructions, the families are briefed on each client brought into their home. This briefing includes the type of medication, if any; the diagnosis in lay terms; the treatment plan; and any special instructions specific to the client, such as people who may come to visit, special diet needs, and the like.

The home sponsors are visited daily by the home coordinators to see that all is going well and to provide information to the sponsor. In addition, each day clients are visited in the homes by their therapist. At this time the home sponsor is interviewed by the therapist to gain information concerning the client's stay. One clinician told us that the home sponsors were the source of much valuable information about the clients because "they will tell them [the home sponsors] things they won't tell us in a clinical interview." The home is also visited at least twice each week by the medical director. Thus, supervision and evaluation of the client take place on a daily basis, and the information gained is fed back to the home sponsors on a regular basis.

The Tollard family of Denver was the first family to receive a client five years ago. They have continued as home sponsors ever since. According to them, responsibility and availability of staff members from the center is the key to the program's success and the reason why they have remained with the program so long. According to Mr. Tollard, "We can count on backup from the center. I know that at any time, day or night, I can call and there will be someone here within 15 minutes." He went on to say, "we probably wouldn't last 24 hours [as home sponsors] if we couldn't count on the backup."

Clients frequently receive psychotropic medication while they are in sponsors' homes. The medical director explains that about 75% of the clients in the alternative homes receive medication. She further stated: "The criteria are no different for medications here than in a 24-hour facility. . . . If they need to be on medication, they are on medication. If not, they are not." The rapid tranquilization procedure does not occur frequently.

The reactions of most of the neighbors to the alternative homes can be generalized first as cautious concern and then as gradual acceptance. Community residents in southwest Denver generally were not notified in advance that there would be an alternative home for psychiatric patients in their neighborhood. Home sponsors maintained a low profile and gradually informed their neighbors about the program as it gained credibility. Mental health education in the neighborhood was enhanced by the kind of trusting relationship sponsors had with their neighbors before the program began. That trust seems to play a significant part in the reduction of neighbors' fears of psychiatric patients and gradual acceptance of individuals with problems.

Clients spend an average of 10 days in the alternative home placements. The community social system awaiting a client influences the length of stay. For example, if there is a delay in getting a job or in getting welfare payments to finance relocation into a private apartment or a boarding home, more time will be spent in the alternative home.

While the clients are in the homes they often help with shopping, meal preparation, household chores, or yardwork. By the time they leave the family, friendships have frequently started to form. Clients often maintain contact with their home sponsors through phone calls, letters, or informal visits. For clients with limited support systems, alternative families provide a base from which they can gain strength both during and after their home placement.

The Tollard family has a collection of several small gifts given to them by clients over the past five years. One was a small set of ceramic salt and pepper shakers inscribed: "My house is small, No mansion for a millionaire; But there is room for love and friends, And that's all I care." Another gift was a board on which a client glued a piece of string to spell "Thank You."

Use of Paraprofessionals

Paraprofessionals are found in a variety of roles at the Southwest Denver center, including home sponsors, administrative personnel, and clinicians. Paraprofessionals fill 14 of the 17 direct service clinician positions. The types of responsibilities a clinician has and the kinds of activities engaged in are directly related to that person's abilities, skills, and interests. These factors are viewed as much more relevant to successful task performance than is the amount of formal education a clinician has obtained.

When professional staff members were asked about the advantages of using paraprofessionals, the following responses were given: "They speak the same language; they relate [to the clients]"; "They have life experiences in common [with the clients]"; "Pragmatic orientation"; "They don't let theoretical categories get in the way"; "They don't have a competing theoretical framework"; "Openness to training"; "They do a lot of things a professional would not like to do."

The overriding comments suggest that the paraprofessionals and professionals are complementary and that this combination of talents renders better service than either could render alone.

Recruitment and Selection

The recruitment and hiring of SWDCMHS personnel is the responsibility of the appropriate program managers and the line supervisors. Employees are informed of the job openings and given preferences in the selection process. If no current employee is qualified, the vacancy is advertised publicly. At present a center priority is to reach qualified racial minorities with an emphasis on Chicano applicants because of the large number of Chicano persons in the center's catchment area.

All hiring committees include a paraprofessional member. Ethnic background is given high priority in the formation of these committees as a means of carrying out the center's affirmative action policies. Each hiring committee designates its own committee chairperson, who may be a paraprofessional staff member. The selection criteria for applicants seem to be: a compatible philosophical position with the center on community mental health work; the ability of the individuals to perceive their own areas of weakness, admit them, and seek out help to eliminate them; an interest in the community; and the willingness and ability to share personal experiences such as those which come from a particular ethnic background. An additional requirement was noted in a comment from the manager of the Adult Psychiatry Services Program: "I wouldn't take a fresh [inexperienced] *anyone* if I could help it; we want experience."

Training

Recruits learn primarily on the job, although there is some inservice training (biweekly), and some release time for personnel to upgrade abilities through workshops, classes, exchanges with other centers, consulting, and conferences. A minimum of 40 hours a year of training outside the center is recommended (80 hours maximum), and this activity is considered to be part of the job.

In practice, the training procedure involves the new clinicians' adapting to a method of service delivery that is compatible with the philosophy of the center. This means training the new staff members to work in the social systems in the community. This service delivery approach demands a high level of autonomy, independence, and the ability to manage the high level of anxiety inherent in "knocking on a door and really not knowing exactly what to expect." On-the-job training at the center is an ongoing procedure and does not terminate at the end of any specific time. Training and upgrading of skills continues by means of supervision and evaluation.

Through a buddy system the trainees are included in situations with many different, experienced clinicians. The key to the successful operation of this system is that the trainees are encouraged to identify and report their areas of weakness, insecurity, and ignorance. They are then paired with a buddy, or several buddies, to work on these areas. Trainees gradually take on more active roles until the buddies, the supervision group, and the supervisor feel they are competent to work with only the normal support and supervision.

Supervision

Southwest Denver Community Mental Health Services, Inc., invests a lot of energy and time in supervision. A supervision group meets weekly and is composed of seven or eight clinicians and a group leader. The group leader is usually a program manager. In this meeting, each clinician presents an ongoing case which provides material useful for group learning. The staff discuss general case problems, as well as those unique to each member's specific area of weakness, so the group may provide help in problem-solving. Each week there is also a meeting involving all the clinicians, where more general clinical and administrative concerns are attended to.

Individual supervision of the clinicians is done by the supervision group leader and by Alice Jones, the paraprofessional program manager of Emergency and Intake, who acts as a troubleshooter in the problem cases which occur.

The medical clinic is held twice weekly. Each client using medication is seen by the medical director and clinician each time a change in medication occurs. The clinician is expected to have knowledge of the medications and make recommendations to the medical director concerning each client. This system provides the clinician with feedback on diagnosis and therapy decisions from the medical director, a psychiatrist; it also provides the medical director a means with which to evaluate the performance of each clinician. The medical director reported that she generally trusts the clinicians' judgments and that building trust is based on the good decisions made by the clinicians. "If I can't trust them [the clinicians], then I really can't do my job," she said.

One of the most important aspects of supervision is that it too is on an informal, daily basis. There are no individual, private offices for clinicians or supervisors, so all nontherapy work is done in a common work room. According to one staff member: "Not having offices contributes to the level of daily supervision; the interaction occurs because you see each other."

Mobility

The philosophy of the center is that the only limit to the paraprofessional staff member's mobility is competence and the legal requirements for the job. The job descriptions for the center have degree requirements for the positions of executive director, the medical director, and the nurses, which were established by the community board of directors. All other clinical and administrative positions specify only skill criteria. Functionally, however, there is very little job mobility. All the administrative or management positions, with the exception of Alice Jones, are held by professionals. The feeling of the paraprofessional staff members who were interviewed was that the possibility for mobility was slight because very few people leave the center, and in reality an advanced degree is necessary for promotion from a clinician to a management or administrative position.

In the Adult Psychiatry Services Program, the clinician series has four levels with separate job descriptions, but in practice only the middle two levels are used. Clinician I is designed for someone with very limited experience, and has never been filled. Clinician II is for persons considered to be in their training period, at the end of which they are promoted to clinician III. Clinician IV exists only on paper, and no one had ever been promoted to fill this slot. The mobility, therefore, is limited to the clinician III level and seems to be a primary concern of the paraprofessional staff. In the words of one of the paraprofessional clinicians, "I just wish there was a clinician III-and-a-half or something."

The clinicians feel that job mobility exists theoretically, but only if "someone dies," because one result of working at an excellent center such as SWDCMHS is that no one leaves. So, most of the paraprofessional clinicians find themselves dead-ended at the clinician III job level with no way to expand except in competence and skills. As one clinician put it, "I put my energy into my work" (instead of into vertical mobility).

There is no arbitrary limit to horizontal mobility and opportunity for innovation within existing structures. The paraprofessional staff members feel there is a great deal of latitude to explore new ideas such as developing a three-quarters way house for clients who need only very minor supervision and help getting started in the community; organizing a men's group, a divorce group, and a mothers' support group; and arranging for a *curandera* folk healer who would be directly responsive to certain client needs in the Chicano community. The only limits to innovation are financial and the clinician's time and energy. There are only so many activities that can be performed in a 40-hour week.

Status and Morale

Status appears to be based upon performance, competence, innovation, and a willingness to share special competencies. The elimination of private offices in favor of a common work room and shared rooms for therapy eliminates one major area for seeking status. Dr. Polak is a good example of the SWDCMHS attitude toward status. His executive office is extremely small and sparsely furnished with a small table and three canvas director's chairs. When he was asked about his less-than-prestigious office he replied: "I have a high opinion of *myself* and regard all the trappings as bullshit. I get my kicks from creating alternatives." This attitude seems to permeate the staff members, both in their image of themselves and their relations to each other.

When a paraprofessional staff member was asked why the center is so successful she responded: "What makes it happen? Me! I count; I am somebody; my decisions are listened to. They may not be bought, but I am heard."

In terms of service delivery and pride in the center and its approach to community mental health, the morale is very high, as reflected in the previous statement and recurrent phrases such as: "We can count on support," and "We have backup."

Evaluation

Evaluation is an ongoing daily and weekly process carried out through the supervision structure already discussed. In addition, the results of formal periodic reviews become part of the clinician's personnel file. The first review takes place three months after the person is hired and occurs annually thereafter. The criteria for evaluation are the job description and the clinician's procedural knowledge, personal functioning, medical knowledge, set of personal growth goals established with the supervisor the year before, and feedback from clients as to the perceived quality of the treatment received. It appears that the clients are very pleased with the treatment they receive from the paraprofessional clinicians.

For evaluation, the clinician, in consultation with the supervisor, prepares a list of 10 clients, community persons, and staff who will evaluate the clinician's performance for the previous year. The criterion for choosing the persons is simply to choose those persons who know the clinician's work the best. The supervisor—in some cases, with the clinician—then compiles the responses and presents the evaluation in a special supervision group for that purpose. The group makes comments on the clinician's evaluated performance and suggests growth goals for the following year. The results of the evaluation procedure are taken into consideration in determining salary, and also can be used to determine probation or termination for a staff member.

In Conclusion

Paraprofessional staff members are integral to the services provided by the Southwest Denver Community Mental Health Center. The manager of emergency services is a paraprofessional whose responsibilities include program administration and clinical supervision; 14 of the 17 clinician positions are staffed by paraprofessionals, who provide crisis, outpatient, and inpatient therapy; the home sponsors are average community families who are paid to open their homes to clients who would otherwise need to be hospitalized. Paraprofessional staff members are ideally suited to the innovative delivery of services provided at the Southwest Denver center particularly because of their lack of commitment to more traditional modes of treatment.

Chapter 9

FOLLOW-UP SERVICES

INTRODUCTION

Description of the Service Area

Community mental health centers are required to provide follow-up care on a voluntary basis for catchment district residents who have been discharged from a public mental health facility. This service was mandated originally by the 1975 Community Mental Health Center Amendments. While most members of the client population are former residents of state mental hospitals, this population also includes persons who have been discharged from inpatient wards at mental health centers and from various residential and transitional facilities.

While the first responsibility of the mental health center is to provide continuing mental health treatment as needed, the follow-up program should also consider the individualized needs of each client for medical care, work or other daily activities, adequate living arrangements, or recreation. Because follow-up services should maximize the capacity of the client to function independently within the community, follow-up service personnel should both establish and maintain contact with their clients. It is desirable that one person provide continuity of care through a set of advocacy, referral, and treatment services for clients. Ideally the relationship between the staff member and client would be a caring one that by itself may contribute to client rehabilitation. The various service components of the mental health center can provide some of the needed services (e.g., day care, consultation services to nursing home staff members, and psychosocial rehabilitation). Volunteers, concerned community citizens, and former patients as well, can be involved in efforts to provide for the needs of follow-up clients. A follow-up program optimally establishes and maintains cooperative relationships both with relevant state mental health facilities and various community agencies that can provide needed service to clients. In addition to the following case study, the interested reader may wish to refer to the chapters covering transitional services and day care services, which contain descriptions of programs that overlap somewhat with this service area.

Selection of the Site Visited

The recommendations for follow-up programs were provided by regional Health, Education, and Welfare offices, as well as by one specialist within the National Institute of Mental Health in Washington, D. C. All seven of the programs surveyed provide follow-up care to patients discharged from state mental hospitals; about one-half of these programs also provide services to patients discharged from the center's inpatient ward. It is rare for services to be provided to discharged clients from other types of organizations, such as community-based residential drug treatment agencies.

While follow-up services are often comprehensive and multifaceted in scope, two structural factors often interfere with the efficacy of follow-up programs. First, the relationship between the follow-up programs and the state hospital(s) often is not a close and collaborative one, either because of the great distance (e.g., 150 miles) separating the two organizations or because of a reported lack of desire to cooperate by state hospital staff members. As a result, follow-up staff members do not typically work with patients or with state hospital staff on predischarge planning for patients. Follow-up services are limited, secondly, by the fact that some mental health centers (and/or communities) do not provide the discharged patients with residential alternatives to private nursing homes. In these instances, follow-up staff make do by referring the discharged patients who lack suitable private living arrangements to the best available nursing homes in the catchment district.

The programs surveyed employ from one to 35 paraprofessionals; the majority of paraprofessionals are B.A. level. Paraprofessionals are always involved in outreach services (e.g., helping patients to find housing; acting as advocates and ombudspersons with public agencies) and are often involved in treatment planning. In about one-third of the programs paraprofessionals lead activity groups or provide group or individual counseling services. Because paraprofessionals who have past experience in follow-up programs are uncommon, the programs surveyed train paraprofessionals in relevant follow-up skills. Some program administrators reported trying to hire paraprofessionals with previous experience working in inpatient wards and with the ability to make decisions autonomously while on outreach assignments.

The follow-up program of the Cambridge-Somerville Community Mental Health and Retardation Center was highly recommended by the Boston HEW regional office. It meets the requirements of federal guidelines and provides a number of additional features. Each paraprofessional at Cambridge-Somerville works continuously with an individual client from the time the client is admitted to the neighboring state hospital to the time that the discharged client no longer needs or chooses to receive follow-up services. The services include predischarge planning with patients in the hospital setting. In addition, the paraprofessionals receive excellent training and supervision from highly skilled professionals, with a dual focus on relevant clinical and social work skills and on the subtleties of establishing a close but professional relationship with clients. Accordingly, clients at Cambridge-Somerville receive (unless a staff paraprofessional resigns) long-term continuity of care in the context of a caring relationship. The paraprofessionals provide a wide variety of diagnostic, outreach, treatment, and advocacy services and have helped to initiate programs that otherwise would not be available to clients. In addition, the follow-up staff members maintain close collaborative ties with other programs within the mental health center and with various public agencies and community organizations.

Cambridge-Somerville Mental Health & Retardation Center: A Case Study in Follow-up Services*

The Cambridge-Somerville Mental Health and Retardation Center serves the 190,000 (1970 census) residents of Cambridge and Somerville, Massachusetts. The center contains 12 programs for children and adults. There is no centralized facility, and the center's programs are located throughout the community. All center programs make extensive use of paraprofessionals in the delivery of services.

The Ambulatory Community Services (ACS) program of the center is an aftercare service that assists patients returning from the Westboro State Hospital in making the transition from the hospital back into the community 35 miles away. This assistance, in fact, is provided from the time the patients are

*Contact: Cambridge-Somerville Mental Health and Retardation Center
        Cambridge Hospital
        1493 Cambridge Street
        Cambridge, Massachusetts   02139
        617/354-2020, ext. 563-564
        Attention: Paul G. Cotton, Nina Marlowe, Program Directors, Ambulatory Community Services

admitted to the hospital. The program provides services to former hospital patients in the areas of alcoholism, drug abuse, mental retardation, outpatient therapy, and day treatment. The ACS paraprofessionals, who prefer to be called ACS workers, provide a link for those patients who are attempting to make the transition from hospital to community life.

The workers spend two days each week in the hospital, and the remaining time in the community at various agency facilities and on community assignments. In providing the linkage services, the paraprofessionals help patients to choose among a variety of community-based services, and then remain available as resource persons to patients and programs to which patients have been referred. Patients are assisted in making contact with appropriate public agencies, such as the welfare department; and with other resources, such as a community-created cooperative apartment association and with the services developed by the ACS program especially for patients discharged from the hospital. Paraprofessionals in the ACS program are directly supervised by the center's clinically-oriented professionals, who help them to provide community-based services that are appropriate to the patients' clinical needs. This multicomponent role demands a much higher level of skill from the ACS paraprofessionals than working in more traditional aftercare referral services.

Background

The Cambridge-Somerville Center was established in 1969 and is funded by a variety of city, state, and federal sources. It operates on an annual budget of $6,400,000 and employs about 190 paraprofessionals and 240 professionals in service roles.

Cambridge-Somerville is a diverse catchment district, containing a mix of the transient poor, stable lower-middle class families, and students and employees of two prestigious universities (Harvard and the Massachusetts Institute of Technology). The very considerable collaboration between the center and the many organizations within the community is a response to this diversity.

The center has strong ties with a number of community agencies and a close working relationship with an area board comprised of community citizens. The center has also recruited Harvard personnel as consultants to and trainees in its program. The Cambridge-Somerville wards of the Westboro State Hospital were incorporated as a center program in July 1973.

In 1972, the State Legislature passed a bill freeing 26 Westboro State Hospital positions for use by a hospital located closer to Cambridge and Somerville. However, when the legislature discovered that 50 additional positions would be required by such a service, it made plans to return the positions to the Westboro State Hospital. Acting quickly, the center director, Dr. Robert C. Reid, drafted overnight a plan for the ACS Program. The legislature allowed the 26 positions to be assigned to the center.

Dr. Paul Cotton was hired by Dr. Reid to implement the ACS Program. Previously, Dr. Cotton had done some work in a community-based aftercare service as a part of his residency training at the Tufts New England Medical Center in Boston. A steering committee was formed during the spring of 1973 to plan the ACS Program. The committee included Dr. Reid, Dr. Cotton, and the directors of the component center programs that would be collaborating with the ACS Program. The ACS Program began on July 1, 1973. Paul Cotton has remained with the ACS Program since its inception. Dr. Nina Marlowe joined him as codirector in July 1975.

Dr. Cotton very deliberately established close working relationships with the Westboro Hospital director and with the particular hospital staff members (the social workers) who would be most directly involved in the discharging of patients back into the community. Also, Dr. Cotton spent considerable time at the hospital participating in meetings, asking hospital staff about their needs, and just talking to hospital employees. The result was a good working relationship with the hospital, which has enabled Dr. Cotton to make the ACS Program acceptable to the hospital.

The ACS Program hired some of the hospital staff as ACS workers, thus smoothing over distinctions between the two programs. In addition, the hospital was reorganized into neighborhood-based wards, containing patients from community neighborhoods rather than patients who shared either a common diagnosis or the same level of functional impairment.

The ACS workers focused first on building a strong working relationship with the hospital staff; they did so by jointly defining deliberately vague ACS roles. As part of this process, the workers solicited ideas from the hospital staff members instead of criticizing current hospital procedures. But the ACS workers also influenced the role of the hospital staff members, primarily by tactfully introducing new ideas and issues at biweekly ward meetings.

The ACS Program operates on an annual budget of $172,000 (supplemented by $25,000 in state hospital funds for one full-time psychiatrist position, shared equally by the two codirectors). The 14 ACS workers receive annual salaries ranging from $7,900 to $8,500. The three R.N.s receive $11,000 annually. The B.A. level program administrator receives $7,900 annually. In addition, the program employs one full-time researcher (B.A. level) who receives an annual salary of $7,900. The program receives $6,600 for travel expenses to and from the Westboro State Hospital.

Program Organization and Services

The ACS Program is organized within the hospital to provide a *focus for discharge.* The neighborhood-based ACS teams can collaborate with and support hospital ward employees interested in discharge planning. Each patient admitted can be helped in discharge planning by as many as three or four ACS staff. These ACS staff members are the two paraprofessionals assigned to each neighborhood-based ward; one of two program nurses, each responsible for two or more wards; and a paraprofessional specializing in geriatric cases. An alcoholism ward has two paraprofessionals and a full-time nurse, all specializing in alcoholism cases. Each nurse has primary responsibility in the work setting for the paraprofessionals and for patients under her jurisdiction. The nurses in turn are each responsible to the program codirectors.

The program B.A. level administrator plays the key role of requiring the ACS staff members to log in their whereabouts and of referring phone calls from clients to the appropriate ACS workers. The administrator also maintains files on all patients and employees and posts notices about employment opportunities, free community events, etc., for use by ACS workers and by patients who drop in. The job requires a person who can work under pressure and in chaotic circumstances—the telephone rings constantly.

The ACS workers and nurses provide a wide array of pre- and postdischarge services to about 350 clients annually. During an average year, the program also continues to serve a somewhat larger number of clients discharged during preceding years.

The predischarge services involve planning for posthospital needs and decisions concerning when discharge is appropriate. Each patient is asked to indicate on a checklist the postdischarge services that would be helpful.

The postdischarge services provided by ACS workers are determined partially by the checklist. These services may include linkage with center and community services, including day treatment, vocational rehabilitation, pastoral counseling, and individual or group therapy. ACS workers may also act as assistants to patients in activities such as moving into a cooperative apartment with other patients, applying for general relief, help with landlord problems, help in finding a room or apartment, tracing lost checks, and grocery shopping. Finally, the ACS workers can link patients with an array of services created by the workers to fill patient needs that are unmet by the center or community. These services include an emergency loan fund, a halfway house, medication groups, a drop-in recreational center, and a discussion group.

Evidence that is described later in the *program evaluation* section of this chapter suggests that the ACS Program has contributed to a steadily declining state hospital census. As a result, ACS workers have been able to provide a wider variety of specialized postdischarge services, including one-to-one therapy for clients who can not be referred to normal outpatient services. Workers providing therapy services receive careful supervision from professionals. The former patients receiving therapy from ACS workers can be highly unreliable in keeping appointments, unable to reach an outpatient clinic, or very difficult people with whom to maintain traditional therapeutic dialogues. For these reasons, such people often "fall through the cracks" of outpatient therapy services; without the ACS workers, these patients might not receive any therapy.

The program's major feature is the extended period of continuous care provided to clients. Beginning with predischarge planning, the care by individual ACS workers can continue until discharge clients no longer require assistance. The role requires of ACS workers both an ability to fit into the highly structured hospital and a knack for working autonomously within unstructured community situations. This basic pattern of activities is supplemented by various unique components.

1. Assistance is provided by the "Westboro Advisory Council," a subcommittee board that helps to administer the mental health center. The council consists of "high functioning" former patients (who still receive services from ACS workers), two ACS workers, hospital and center staff, and members of the center's community board. Its task is to focus on improving ACS services to patients. For example, a former patient (and current council member) visited rooming houses available to former patients and compiled a rating list for use by ACS workers and discharged patients. As another example, the council is developing a booklet to guide discharged patients in welfare, housing, and other relevant areas of concern. The committee also runs fund-raising drives to finance new services, such as a drop-in center, needed by former patients.

2. A special team in the hospital works in a ward for alcoholics and occasional drug-abuse patients. This arrangement enables the patients to see themselves as having drug-related difficulties, rather than as being mentally ill. Because alcoholic patients tend to be male, it is important that at least one ACS alcoholism worker be a male.

3. The "ACS loan fund" is a small ($1,600) grant secured by an ACS worker. The loans are small—averaging $10–$35—but can be very helpful. For example, a loan can provide starter money for a patient who cannot receive welfare until he or she has moved into a community residence. Or a loan can help a discharged patient pay for basic living expenses when a welfare or disability check has failed to arrive on time.

4. ACS workers have established a drop-in center in Cambridge and are currently establishing one in Somerville. The Cambridge facility is located in the basement of a church, at some distance from other center services, and provides discharged patients with a clublike setting for social and recreational activities. For clients who do not need or wish to receive day treatment services, the drop-in center provides an alternative to sitting at home. For clients receiving day treatment, the drop-in center provides a treatment-free place for relaxation and socialization. Activities at the drop-in center include a body movement group, ping pong, television watching, bake sales, and occasional outings to the countryside.

5. In a side room of the currently established drop-in center, nurses lead medication groups. These groups promote attendance at the drop-in cen-

ter by giving people an "excuse for coming." Simultaneously, the location of medication groups at drop-in centers causes patients to feel relaxed about coming to receive their drugs, and enables the program staff members to maintain ongoing contact with their clients.

Program Evaluation.   The program has been evaluated by a recent "consumer satisfaction" study conducted by the ACS staff researcher. This self-evaluation effort, funded by the ACS Program itself, involved a series of one-to-one structured interviews between the ACS researcher and the client-participants. Clients were invited to participate both orally and through letters. The 22 client participants were all actively receiving ACS services at the time of participation, and were selected by their expressing an interest in being involved in the survey. The questionnaire schedule, constructed for the purpose of the self-study, has not been examined for reliability or validity features.

The data gathered by the permanent ACS staff researcher strongly support the hypothesis that ACS services help to increase the period of community stay by discharged patients and to decrease the number of problems experienced during the postdischarge period. Because the services are primarily delivered by ACS workers, the data also bear on the effectiveness of paraprofessionals. The data, however, do not prove conclusively that ACS services cause these effects, for the information was not gathered from a controlled study comparing patients receiving and not receiving ACS services.

The census of the Cambridge-Somerville Hospital ward has steadily declined from about 325 in July 1973 to about 100 in January 1977. Many of the current patients are severe "chronics" or alcoholics who repeatedly return from community stays. Currently, about 50 to 60% of discharge patients are readmitted at some future date. The census reduction probably reflects a combination of ACS efforts and pressures upon and within the hospital to reduce its population.

A past history of alcoholism is the strongest predictor of return to the hospital by discharged patients. The return rate of all other discharged patients is about 25%. Why is the ACS service not more effective with alcohol-prone clients? One factor may be the nature of the disease. Alcoholism is not easily cured. Another factor involves the ambiguous position of clients with a dual diagnosis of previous alcoholism and previous psychosis. Some discharged dual diagnosis patients probably require structured living situations designed for persons with their particular history. Neither the center nor the program has been able to secure funding for such specialized halfway house settings.

Two factors directly related to ACS services also predict the length of community stay by discharged patients. The more areas in which aftercare services (e.g., housing) are provided to discharged patients, the longer the patient remains in the community. The period of community stay also increases with the number of aftercare areas covered by the predischarge planning process.

The number of problems (e.g., difficulty with money) experienced during community stays decreases with the number of areas (e.g., welfare) covered in predischarge planning. The number of problems experienced by discharged clients also decreases with the number of aftercare contacts from ACS workers.

The ACS researcher also considered client satisfaction with specific ACS postdischarge services. The clients indicated that the "most helpful" ACS function involved the personal relationship (e.g., "talking to my ACS worker") with the ACS worker. Thus, the client-worker relationship appears to be a particularly important component of the ACS Program.

Finally, discharged patients were asked to choose the person they would contact in future times of trouble. Possible choices included hospital staff, ACS staff, relatives, friends, and professionals from center or community agencies. About 50% of the respondents indicated their ACS worker as a first choice.

Use of Paraprofessionals

The program does not employ the term "paraprofessional." Rather, B.A. and sub-B.A. staff members are called "ACS workers" and are considered to be "professionals without a discipline." An ACS worker is a person who helps a former patient to become established in the community—through planning services, assistance in carrying out tasks, and provision of emotional support. The ACS workers provide competent services at a low cost. In addition, they effectively carry out strenuous tasks that many professional workers don't wish to do.

A B.A. level researcher keeps records for the program. She gathers patient admission and discharge statistics, and charts how the staff members spend their time. Furthermore, the researcher is responsible for conducting any client interviews that go beyond the direct clinical needs of the clients. She presents information in easy-to-understand charts that enable ACS staff members to gain an overview of their activities. It is her research that indicates the importance of the ACS worker's most essential activity—maintenance of a good relationship between the individual ACS worker and the clients.

The ACS workers claim that good relationships with clients are established through a consistent set of efforts that convince the clients that the worker truly cares about them and their welfare. By becoming involved in both the daily and extraordinary service needs of clients, the ACS workers communicate the attitude that clients are people to them rather than a "bundle of problems." Such services may include a range of assistance on routine tasks, such as shopping at the grocery store or paying daily visits to a patient who is hospitalized for medical care; or more complicated advocacy services, such as helping to untangle complications with the Department of Welfare; and on extra services such as picking up something from the home of a patient who is currently at the hospital.

As ACS workers establish close and trusting relationships with their clients, it becomes more and more likely that they will be asked for advice. Such advice is usually given "on the run," while ACS workers are helping clients with daily living matters. The ACS workers are encouraged by their clinical supervisors to provide such counseling within clear limits and under careful supervision.

The supervisors teach ACS workers to make a distinction between "secondary" and "primary" process thinking. Secondary process thinking is objective and reality oriented—e.g., "How do I meet people?" Primary process thinking is symbolic and related to complicated themes involving the inner life of the client—e.g., "Why is everyone against me?" ACS workers are encouraged to discuss secondary process issues with clients and when primary process issues arise, to shift the focus to more objective issues. Thus, the workers do not become involved in clinical issues that exceed their competence.

When it is possible, the workers are guided by their supervisors to speak with their clients about these practical problems and to help clients by offering concrete suggestions, such as explaining some of the services the center can provide. For example, an ACS worker will offer to take a client concerned about how to meet people to the program's drop-in center. Or the worker may gently persuade a client who has become overdependent to take a first step by venturing to the grocery store alone.

Recently, some ACS workers have been setting aside scheduled blocks of time for talking with clients about issues that concern them. The issues discussed and the guidelines followed parallel those that would be otherwise discussed on the run. These sessions, however, can delve somewhat more deeply into issues. The ACS workers receive individualized supervision from professional clinicians, whether counseling informally or during scheduled blocks of time. Another important aspect of training for this sensitive type of work consists of the psychotherapy seminars which all workers take prior to becoming involved in more formalized one-to-one therapy relationships with clients.

There are occasions when a worker develops a new service as a need is recognized. For example, one ACS worker, with supervision from a professional, supplements her regular ACS duties by providing group therapy to families of patients who are to be discharged from the hospital. The families meet weekly in groups that provide an accepting atmosphere for discussion of matters of common concern, such as the guilt that many feel for having perhaps contributed in some way to a patient's institutionalization. It is important to dispel these feelings by talking them out *before* the patient is discharged, lest the family members take on too many of the newly discharged patient's responsibilities and interfere with the essential process of regaining independence and self-respect.

One important aspect of follow-up care for discharged patients is the establishment of a good relationship between the ACS worker and the welfare or Supplementary Security Income (SSI) case worker. After a good relationship is established, the ACS worker can call the case worker to make minor requests. Also, the ACS worker often accompanies the patient on visits to the welfare or SSI office, after having made an appointment in advance. The personal presence of the ACS worker can be beneficial to frightened patients or to patients who might claim unrealistically that they are able to work. By being present, the ACS worker can also help the case worker with a possibly difficult client.

One ACS worker is a full-time specialist on cooperative apartment living. She collaborates with the local community group that began cooperative living units for people who need supervision but not a live-in staff. Of the three program apartments, two are for women, and one is for men. Each apartment accommodates four or five residents. This ACS worker locates and manages the apartments, selects applicants for the apartments, runs groups that prepare patients for cooperative apartment living, leads meetings of residents to discuss routine matters and crisis situations, acts as a liaison between the program and the community group responsible for the apartments, does public relations work for the local organization, and collaborates with the ACS workers assigned to the former patients who live in the apartments.

Certain individual ACS workers specialize in providing services to ex-alcoholic and to geriatric clients. The members of the alcoholism team work with a very difficult-to-help population of clients. In order to avoid feelings of personal incompetence, the workers attempt to set low expectations for themselves. Clients with dual psychosis-alcoholism diagnoses require more emotional support and task assistance than do alcoholic clients. Thus, the ACS alcoholism workers make special efforts to establish a personal relationship with discharged patients and to communicate very clearly to them their sincere willingness to provide assistance upon request. Discharged patients from the alcoholism ward have a special need for financial support, for they typically are not able to work for some time. Thus, the ACS workers make efforts to arrange special loans and rapid processing of welfare and other payments for these clients. Before discharge, patients on the alcoholism ward participate in a special ACS-led group that focuses on issues related to both alcoholism and psychosis.

Most geriatric patients in the hospital are referred by nursing homes, and discharged geriatric clients generally return to nursing homes. Thus, the ACS geriatric workers have developed skills for working with nursing home staff as well as with elderly clients.

It is important that the ACS workers see elderly clients as individuals, rather than as stereotyped old people. Because geriatric clients frequently wish to talk about death and dying, the ACS workers receive some training in dealing with these topics. Older clients may have impaired abilities to hear, see, remember, and learn. If appropriate, the ACS workers speak to geriatric clients slowly and loudly, being careful not to introduce very many new ideas on any one occasion.

ACS workers increase their impact by developing good relationships with nursing home staff. ACS-nursing home relationships are developed in large measure through consultation and education services that focus on problems of personal importance to staff members.

The following example illustrates how an ACS worker used a consultation contact to improve his working relationship with nursing home staff, and prevented the inappropriate hospitalization of a nursing home resident. A program M.D. suggested and closely supervised the strategy employed by the ACS worker.

A nursing home employee contacted the ACS Program about a resident who was wandering around at night and starting arguments with the night staff. The nursing home staff believed that the previously hospitalized elderly resident required rehospitalization. The ACS geriatric worker who had previously worked with this patient made an appointment to come to the nursing home. The ACS worker first asked the nursing home staff to define the problem from their point of view. The staff described the symptoms of the resident and their annoyance at the behavior. The ACS worker checked the resident's record for clues and discovered that the resident's Valium dosage had recently been increased. Explaining to the nursing home staff that Valium can induce sleep during the day and wakefulness and confusion at night, the ACS worker suggested that the Valium dosage be reduced during the day.

The ACS workers supplement consultation services with educational programs for nursing home staff members. Educational topics have included types of mental disorders, psychological assessment procedures useful with the elderly, appropriate medication procedures for psychological problems, symptoms indicating the presence of undesirable medical side effects, and physical causes for psychological problems.

Recruitment and Selection

The program does not actively recruit applicants. ACS workers are selected from a pool of applications that have been submitted to the program or the center. Some applicants are state hospital employees who are familiar with the ACS Program. Previous work in inpatient treatment settings is a valuable background experience. However, it is even more important that applicants be able to relate well to clients and to fellow ACS workers. Applicants must be able to tolerate frustratingly slow progress by clients in an unstructured community-based work setting. Clinical skills are helpful, but they can be taught after the worker is selected. Thus, applicants that can relate well to other people and can work autonomously are sometimes chosen in preference to applicants with considerable clinical training and/or work experience.

An applicant's ability to relate to other people is assessed through interviews by a program codirector and by members of the team to which the applicant would be assigned. Reactions of prospective colleagues are a very important consideration in hiring decisions. In addition, the applicant may be asked to discuss family background. Generally, applicants with happy family experiences are seen as lower-risk candidates.

Applicants hired by the ACS Program are usually in their twenties, with social science B.A. or B.S. degrees. They did not necessarily grow up within the catchment district, nor do they all live there. Dr. Cotton, the ACS Program codirector, has worked in another successful aftercare program that used workers without college degrees, and emphasizes that a group of sub-B.A. level catchment area residents could work effectively.

Training

New ACS workers require about three months of training before developing the skills required to work autonomously in the community. The new workers are told that this period of adjustment is normal and that they have permission to say "no" to demands that seem excessive to them.

The orientation provided by the ACS Program primarily involves meeting with various staff members on a one-to-one basis. Initially, the new staff members are provided with a written description of the ACS procedures, services, the center, and the community resources. Then, the new employee meets with the staff experts, many of whom are ACS workers, for separate 60- to 90-minute meetings on specific topics. Training in clinical skills entails several individual hour-long meetings with one of the program codirectors. These sessions focus on intake and diagnostic procedures, strategies for recognizing and handling client life crises, formulation of discharge plans, and assessment of when a patient is ready for discharge.

Each new staff member receives training from the center's alcoholism program. Alcoholism is a common problem in the catchment district and is frequently encountered by ACS workers.

Also offered to all newly hired nurses and paraprofessionals is a core curriculum orientation training program. This training program prevents duplication of orientation procedures by the various center programs, and attendance is required. Thus, program directors cannot divert new employees from these sessions by requiring that they attend to pressing service delivery needs. The eight topics covered by the center orientation program are interlaced with discussions of appropriate therapeutic relationships with the clients, often based on true case histories. These discussions highlight the risks involved in extending a helping relationship to the level of friendship or romance.

The new ACS worker is paired with a buddy who acts as a peer tutor. The buddy is another ACS worker from the new employee's team or else the nurse whose responsibilities include the given team. The new employee gradually shifts from watching, to acting while being observed, to carrying out responsibilities with increasing autonomy.

In-service Training.   All new ACS workers are required to attend weekly center lectures during their first year of employment. These lectures cover many topics and are aimed simultaneously at professional and paraprofessional audiences. Furthermore, all ACS workers (no matter how long employed) must attend one center seminar each semester. In addition, the program offers an ongoing interviewing seminar to ACS staff members.

The ACS workers do not receive academic credit for their work experiences or training. The fact that the ACS workers already have B.A. or B.S. degrees has made it impossible for the center to arrange such credit unless the workers are enrolled in a formal M.A. program.

Supervision

Each ACS worker receives an hour of supervision weekly from two different program professionals. Each year a worker is assigned new supervisors. Thus, ACS workers learn varying perspectives from several professionals.

Supervisors use these meetings to highlight the real progress being made by clients as well as to make suggestions for improvement of services. Aftercare work is demanding and frustrating; the ACS workers require praise as well as constructive criticism. Newly hired ACS workers receive supervision for most of their patients. Supervision of more experienced ACS workers focuses on difficult clients and on crisis situations.

Mobility

According to ACS Program staff, the cost-effectiveness and continuity of care provided by the ACS Program are impaired by the salary restrictions and resulting mobility problems imposed upon the center and program by Massachusetts state employment guidelines. Because of budget restraints, the program cannot afford to pay M.A.-level salaries to people who carry out the nonmedical responsibilities that must be implemented by the program. Thus, ACS workers who obtain M.A. degrees cannot advance within the program or center, and must leave the program in order to carry out similar work elsewhere at higher salary levels.

The typical ACS worker remains with the program for 18 months. Workers quit primarily because of the program's low salaries. Many workers say that they would remain with the program if they could earn higher salaries after obtaining M.A. degrees.

During their period with the program, many ACS workers—with active encouragement from the program codirectors—enroll in a masters degree program. The flexible ACS work schedules allow the ACS workers to attend some classes during the day. Program and center professionals help the ACS workers by writing letters of recommendation to M.A. or Ph.D. programs and to prospective employers of workers who have obtained M.A. degrees. The program thus serves ACS workers as a career stepping stone to higher paying jobs. However, the rapid turnover rate of paraprofessionals also places a burden on the program and center. Training and supervision of new ACS workers involves considerable expense. Federal, state, and local sources pay for direct service delivery costs, but not for the expenses involved in training staff members to deliver effective services. These problems will continue as long as the state of Massachusetts fails to upgrade its salary schedule for paraprofessionals.

One contributing factor to the low salaries is that the program cannot receive third-party payments for services delivered by the ACS workers. In order to receive such payments, the program would be required to hire M.D.s to perform ACS services.

When an ACS worker leaves for a higher paying position, the program and center must train a replacement, and the worker's former clients must learn to relate to a different worker. ACS clients can be very upset when their ACS worker leaves the program, for clients often have difficulty in forming relationships and can interpret the loss of a worker as a personal rejection. Because they can receive higher salaries, the program R.N.s remain with the program for longer periods of time. The presence of R.N.s on the staff thus helps to reduce problems in maintaining continuity of care.

Status and Morale

The ACS workers are uniformly unhappy about their salaries, which are barely adequate to cover daily living expenses in the Cambridge-Somerville area and fail to reflect the grueling and highly skilled nature of their work. The job is a "dead end" situation where rewards cannot be given for assuming additional responsibilities. After an average stay of 18 months, many paraprofessionals quit the ACS program to pursue an M.A., Ph.D., or M.D. degree or a higher paying job. However, ACS workers react very positively to many other aspects of the program.

Job Flexibility.   The ACS workers are required to provide basic client services at the hospital and in the community. Within these limits, however, the workers are able to follow individualized work schedules and to take on additional self-designed work responsibilities. The workers, thus, feel trusted by the codirectors, free to create challenging work situations for themselves, and able to utilize their talents fully.

Peer and Team Relationships.   The ACS workers and nurses as a group form friendships and see one another outside of the work situation. The feelings of closeness are enhanced by the program's policy of having the R.N. team directors spend some of their time carrying out the community-based functions of ACS workers. But the good feelings also result from the fact that it is generally felt that ACS staff members are very likable, approachable people, who are able to communicate well and to accept shortcomings in themselves and in their colleagues. ACS workers repeatedly mentioned how very much they had been helped by peer consultation on work-related problems and anxieties. It is highly probable that this sense of mutual support is a direct asset in confronting the difficulties of a challenging job.

The Relationship with the Program Codirectors.   The ACS workers and nurses feel respected by the program codirectors. The codirectors, in turn, report that they genuinely believe that the ACS staff members are capable people.

The program codirectors show their respect in numerous specific ways. Important issues are considered by the entire staff at weekly meetings. For example, the entire staff was involved in approving the visit to the program by a staff member of the Paraprofessional Utilization Project. The codirectors meet with each team on a weekly basis, in order to maintain personal contact with staff members and discuss the progress of team clients. The codirectors contribute time to one-to-one supervision of the ACS staff, and make themselves available to see staff members about work-related or personal crises. Periodically, the codirectors meet with the R.N.s to keep abreast of the interpersonal dynamics within teams. And the codirectors and staff together attend program parties, potluck suppers, and weddings.

Evaluation of Paraprofessional Performance

Evaluation Form.   The ACS staff and one of the codirectors together have developed a rating form to be used after a worker has been employed for six months, and yearly thereafter. The form is completed by the worker's supervisor, the team leader, the coordinators, and by the actual worker. The items concern the worker's relationship to patients and to staff, and use of educational opportunities and appropriate administrative procedures. Each employee has a feedback session about the evaluation with the program codirectors, and with his/her supervisor and team leader. A worker who has been performing below the program's standards can be fired.

Record Keeping.   ACS workers are required to keep records on patient behavior progress before and following hospital discharge. Because of their hectic schedules, however, not all ACS workers set aside sufficient time for record keeping. When available, these records can enhance the value of supervisory sessions.

In Conclusion

The ACS Program at the Cambridge-Somerville Mental Health and Retardation Center provides services to clients from the time of their admission to the state mental hospital, and these services continue until the clients have been discharged and no longer require assistance in readjusting to their local community. This extended period of continuous care is made possible by the paraprofessional staff members. Paraprofessionals work with clients on a one-to-one basis and provide all appropriate nonmedical services. The paraprofessionals work within a highly structured state hospital setting, as well as autonomously on unstructured community assignments. They possess a wide range of skills, performing such tasks as predischarge planning, teaching of basic living skills to clients, serving as client advocates with public agencies, mediating disputes between clients and landlords, intervening in crisis situations, and (under close supervision from professionals) providing therapy services to clients who would not be served by outpatient facilities. The staff paraprofessionals have designed and implemented several services that otherwise would not have been available for clients. The data gathered by the program's research specialist suggest a high degree of effectiveness both for the program and the activities of the staff paraprofessionals.

Chapter 10

INPATIENT SERVICES

Introduction

Description of the Service Area

Community mental health centers have been required to provide for inpatient services since the passage of the original federal legislation in 1963. These services should be designed to provide a therapeutic environment for persons requiring 24-hour care. The major goal of inpatient services is to provide rapid evaluation and effective treatment of persons with severe emotional disturbances in order to facilitate their return to the community. The proper strategy for achieving this goal is to provide short-term, intensive treatment and/or evaluation in a humane manner that promotes and preserves the dignity of the individual patient.

Selection of the Site Visited

The Mid-Columbia Community Mental Health Center in Richland, Washington, was the site we selected in the area of inpatient services. Our initial survey resulted in a number of possible programs, which all followed a fairly traditional staffing pattern: substantial numbers of paraprofessionals working in teams with registered nurses, with psychiatrists maintaining final treatment responsibility. The Mid-Columbia Center has used paraprofessionals extensively since its inception. The paraprofessionals of the inpatient program have treatment responsibility that involves more than the typical custodial tasks. The treatment philosophy emphasizes the nonmedically oriented aspects of client care including a therapeutic milieu approach, a nonhospital physical environment, problem-oriented rather than diagnostic category treatment records, elimination of electroconvulsive shock therapy (ECT), responsible medication policies, and few involuntary commitments. A screening committee monitors the performance of paraprofessional staff members who provide counseling services, and a professional staff member is always available for tasks that are beyond a paraprofessional's competence.

The center meets all of the Health, Education, and Welfare guidelines in the area of inpatient services and was given a strong recommendation by the regional HEW office in Seattle.

Mid-Columbia Mental Health Center: A Case Study in Inpatient Services*

The inpatient facility discussed in this chapter is located in the Mid-Columbia Mental Health Center in Richland, Washington. The center is a private non-profit corporation serving the residents of Franklin and Benton counties in the southeast central portion of the state of Washington. Three cities—Richland, Pasco, and Kennewick—are located in this area in Washington, where the Columbia and the Snake rivers meet. Each city has a population of approximately 30,000 people which accounts for about 90% of the center's catchment population.

The Mid-Columbia Mental Health Center is a comprehensive center offering a full range of services. In addition to the inpatient program, it offers crisis services; day care services for children, adolescents, adults, and geriatric clients; an outpatient program; and consultation and education services. The center also has programs concerning nursing homes, persons with chemical abuse difficulties, the criminal justice system (including the juvenile court), the mentally retarded, and the local Head Start project, as well as a mental illness prevention program. There is also an outreach satellite center located in Pasco. There are paraprofessional staff members in all of these programs, and seven of the programs are coordinated by paraprofessionals.

The inpatient unit provides short-term hospitalization and milieu therapy for a maximum of 22 clients. The service is given by the unit's 28 employees:

*Contact: Mid-Columbia Mental Health Center
       1175 Gribble
       Richland, Washington   99352
       509/943-9104
       Attention: Mike O'Connell, Center Director

12 paraprofessionals, 8 nurses, and 8 other professionals. The primary day-to-day client care is given by the nurses and the paraprofessionals. The paraprofessional staff members are divided into two categories: mental health technicians and mental health specialists. While both provide direct services to the client, the specialists supervise and train the technicians as well.

Background

Richland, Washington, was founded after World War II as a town to house the people building the Hanford Nuclear Power Plant. In 1958, the General Electric Company, which built the plant, began divesting itself of the management of the city. One result of General Electric's withdrawal was the loss to Richland of the physical and mental health care that the company had previously provided residents of the community. For example, after 1958 most of the General Electric medical staff who provided the mental health services began to leave the area. In response to a mental health needs assessment done in 1961 by a citizen group, the United Way funded a Family Counseling and Mental Health Center to fill part of the mental health need.

Mike O'Connell, M.S.W., the current center director, came to the Richland area in 1962. He engaged in private clinical practice and his concern for the unmet mental health needs of the area led him to join a concerned citizen's group. In 1967 a citizens advisory board formed a nonprofit corporation for the purpose of establishing a community-based treatment center. In 1969 the nonprofit corporation arranged with a local hospital to build a detached mental health inpatient facility which would be part of the hospital and accredited with it, but administered separately. The mental health center was built as an inpatient facility that could provide other services as well.

The inpatient unit was designed to be an open facility. Two members of the original nonprofit corporation, Tess Ward, currently the center's associate director, and Helen Warren, now a paraprofessional therapist on the outpatient staff, visited a number of inpatient facilities including the Fort Logan Hospital and the Southwest Denver Community Mental Health Center[1] to gather ideas during the planning stage.

The original conception was that the unit should be as "nonhospital" as possible. Structurally, ten patient rooms radiate symmetrically around a large living-room-like space. This central living area has couches and overstuffed chairs arranged in conversation areas. It includes a television set, telephone, and kitchen area which are specifically for the clients' use. The client rooms each have two beds and a private bath. The inpatient facility resembles a college dormitory much more than a conventional inpatient ward.

Director Mike O'Connell explains that the logic behind the open facility is to "keep the barriers out," and to encourage more open contact by eliminat-

[1] See Emergency Services chapter.

ing as many physical barriers between people as possible. There are no locks on the doors; there are no chairs in the nursing station. Thus, the staff members are encouraged to spend their time with clients in the living room area rather than behind a glass wall. "The unit was designed this way to put staff in a really strong position to help people. It has its headaches, but I wouldn't have it any other way." He sums up the original philosophy of the center by saying, "We don't want to let a kind of professionalism get in the way of delivering services to the client."

Mike O'Connell has been the director of the center since it opened in 1973. The center from the outset was committed to the use of paraprofessional staff. O'Connell became involved with the use of paraprofessionals in mental health service delivery when he was a Rhodes scholar in England. While pursuing his studies, he worked as a paraprofessional in a family service agency that employed paraprofessional staff. This experience made him aware of the ways in which paraprofessional personnel can make valuable contributions in direct service delivery.

O'Connell's belief in the abilities of paraprofessional personnel is demonstrated by the responsible positions they hold in the organization he directs. Seven of the center's 20 programs are coordinated by paraprofessional staff personnel. In one program, the paraprofessional coordinator has the responsibility for a staff of 16, including 13 professionals, 3 of whom are Ph.D. psychologists.

The center currently employs over 100 people, two-thirds of whom are paraprofessionals, and has an annual budget of over $1,758,000. The center as a whole served about 5,500 clients in 1976.

The catchment population of the inpatient program comes from four disparate sources: the cities of Richland, Pasco, and Kennewick, and the rural portion of the two counties. Kennewick is historically a farming town; Pasco grew up around the railroad and today comprises the majority of the poorer and minority population; Richland is a town that did not exist until after World War II, and its fairly new population tends to be highly educated and to work for the Hanford Nuclear Power Center around which the city was built. The rural portion of the catchment area is made up primarily of small family farms. Thus, as a result of the diversity of the catchment's population, the kinds of needs the center is trying to fill are quite broad.

The catchment population of the center is primarily white; the largest minority population is Hispanic in origin—4% to 6%. (It depends upon the time of year since there is a large population of seasonal workers.) The black minority is about 2% of the catchment population. The largest proportional use of the center is made by the black population.

The inpatient unit is the largest program of the Mid-Columbia Mental Health Center. It occupies a full wing of the center. It employs 28 persons full- and part-time, including 12 paraprofessional staff members (9 mental health technicians, 3 mental health specialists), 8 nurses, and 8 other professionals including 2 part-time Ph.D. clinical psychologists, and 2 half-time psychiatrists (time shared with other center programs).

There is a maximum of 22 beds and last year the center admitted 539 patients. Four hundred of these were voluntary admissions. Sixty were originally involuntary commitments and then were changed to voluntary status. In 1976 the average census of the center was 12.5 clients and the average length of stay was 8.2 days. The high number of transfers to a voluntary status and the shortness of stay is in keeping with the inpatient program philosophy of openness and short-term crisis orientation. O'Connell reports there have been periods of over 6 months without an involuntary hold and that he has spent as long as 6 hours convincing a client to be voluntarily admitted.

The goals of the inpatient facility are directed toward prevention, treatment, and rehabilitation. A quotation from the facility's statement of treatment philosophy reads: "First and foremost, efforts to organize therapeutic services in a community mental health program must be governed by a desire to make services available to as many persons in the community as require them." This policy in practice is described by one of the paraprofessional staff members in the inpatient program. "We don't turn anyone away. We are here for people who need help." Tess Ward, the associate director, says, "We provide services to people regardless of their income and this policy really gets in the way of fiscal policy."

The inpatient unit is a short-term (14 day) crisis-oriented residential unit that focuses on helping the clients gain the necessary resources to get them back into the community as quickly as possible. To quote again from the treatment philosophy: "The goal of treatment is: To provide the patient with enough assistance to help him maintain at least a minimal or improved functioning with decreased subjective difficulties." One of the senior paraprofessionals expressed clearly the center's attitude toward clients: "I believe every person has the ability to change and most people don't know how. My job is to help." Another paraprofessional described the inpatient unit as "not a place where you give up your resources, but a place where you marshal them."

There is a strong emphasis on patients' rights at the center. When admitted, patients are given a statement of their rights and these rights are explained. According to the staff, no medication is forced on the patients who are voluntary residents. Patients participate in their own diagnosis and treatment as much as possible and routinely come to staffing sessions when their cases are being discussed. According to one of the psychiatrists, "Clients sometimes have a much better idea about themselves than we do."

The tone of the center is depicted by the Chinese painting on the center's introductory pamphlet entitled "Friends."

Program Organization and Services

The inpatient facility operates 24 hours a day, 365 days a year. The day is broken into three eight-hour shifts and the staffing of each shift rotates each week. Therefore, each person will work a variety of shifts and will seldom work the same shift for more than a week or two in a row. The staff members are rotated so that communication among the employees remains high. In this way, all the people who work for the inpatient program know each other and learn each others' capabilities.

The greatest staff coverage is provided during the day shift. As is typical of inpatient units, nurses work in teams with paraprofessionals providing treatment to clients under the direction of the center psychiatrists. On all of the shifts there are at least three persons—one nurse and two paraprofessional technicians or specialists—one of whom must be male.

The greater part of the facility's activity also takes place during the day. The two psychologists and the social worker attached to the inpatient unit work at that time. Most decisions regarding diagnosis and treatment are made at two daily staffing sessions. These occur at 8:00 a.m. and late in the afternoon. The day shift is managed by the coordinator of the inpatient unit or her assistant. The responsibility for the evening and night shift is rotated among various staff members. Paraprofessionals and nurses share this responsibility.

In order to provide continuity of care over a 24-hour period, each patient is assigned to a three person primary therapist team composed of mental health specialists, technicians, and nurses. These primary therapists have the majority of contact with the client and an effort is made to have one of them on each eight-hour shift.

All primary therapists are responsible for custodial maintenance of their clients as well as for therapeutic relationships in one-to-one or group settings. It is the goal of the inpatient program for clients to have at least three individual therapy sessions with primary therapists daily. It was reported that between 25 and 50 percent of the paraprofessional psychiatric technician's time is spent in therapeutic contact with clients. The percentage varies with the number of clients in the center at any one time and "the sort of day we are having."

When a client is admitted by a doctor to the inpatient unit, the three primary therapists begin to chart information (i.e., a psychosocial history, etc.) which will eventually lead to a diagnosis and a treatment plan. The team is responsible for gathering data to determine the client's primary problem. This is done by developing what they call a Subject Objective Assessment Plan (SOAP) chart. This chart consists of: a *subjective* account of what the client says about the difficulty; an *objective* statement of behavior; an *assessment* of why the therapist thinks the problem exists; and, finally, a *plan* of action to work out the problem.

The findings that the SOAP chart reveals are discussed with the client's psychiatrist and a treatment plan based upon it is developed at the first staffing session for the client. This staffing session is held within 72 hours of the patient's arrival. Those attending this meeting include the client's psychiatrist, at least one of the primary therapists, and the inpatient social worker. The coordinator of the inpatient unit or her assistant, and any day treatment or outpatient therapists who may become the therapist after the discharge of the client, may also attend. Depending upon his or her level of functioning, the client may also be present at the staffing session.

Decisions about problem identification, diagnosis, treatment strategies, and release plans for the client are discussed at this initial staffing session. These decisions are made by the psychiatrist with substantial input from paraprofessional primary therapists and the other persons present at the staffing session. The center views primary therapists as "the eyes and ears of the psychiatrist." The decisions regarding specific treatment strategies, as well as the over-all therapeutic approach, are then carried out by the primary therapists.

There exists an ongoing schedule of activities for all inpatient clients in which the newly admitted client will share partially or totally, depending upon the nature of his or her individual treatment plan which may add or delete activities. The schedule of a sample day follows:

Tuesday, January 7, 1977

8:00–8:30 a.m.	Breakfast	Dining Room
8:30–8:45 a.m.	Ward Government	Living Room
8:45–9:00 a.m.	Exercise Group	Stage Area
9:00–9:30 a.m.	Environmental Maintenance	I/P Unit
9:30–11:00 a.m.	Group Therapy	Music Room
9:30–11:30 a.m.	Expressive Therapy	Workshop
12:00–1:00 p.m.	Lunch	Dining Room
1:00–3:00 p.m.	Psychodrama	Stage Area
1:00–4:00 p.m.	Expressive Therapy	Workshop
4:00–5:00 p.m.	Free Time	I/P Unit
5:00–6:00 p.m.	Dinner	Dining Room
7:00–9:00 p.m.	Music Group	Music Room
Evening	Activity Group	Flexible

The primary therapists log observations of the effectiveness of the treatment strategies and client progress in each client's SOAP chart. This information is fed back to the psychiatrist in morning staffing sessions held daily in which brief information regarding all clients is exchanged. A formal meeting for each client occurs after each seven days of stay to reexamine in depth each client's case. In these subsequent meetings, diagnoses, client problems, and treatment strategies are reexamined and reformed in the light of input from the primary therapists' observations based upon daily contact with clients.

The inpatient program is evaluated yearly by the funding sources and on an ongoing basis by the administrative committee and a utilization review committee. The administrative committee is composed of the center director, the two codirectors, the financial office, and a paraprofessional staff person from the inpatient program. On a biweekly basis, they review the admission and discharge statistics and financial information. They are also responsible for reviewing and making recommendations concerning the overall effectiveness of the program. The utilization review committee reviews client records, randomly selected, to monitor day-to-day activity of the program.

Use of Paraprofessionals

The reasons for using paraprofessionals are varied. One of the first reported is cost. The coordinator of the inpatient program estimates that costs would increase by at least $10,000 to $12,000 a month if paraprofessionals weren't used. This would increase the budget by about 40%. The coordinator of the inpatient program reported, "Without paraprofessionals there would be very little or no therapy." Another professional staff member said, "Without our skilled paraprofessionals it would be little more than a maintenance unit."

There are reasons other than cost however, for employing paraprofessional staff. According to virtually all of the professional staff interviewed, paraprofessionals bring a "freshness of vision" that is very valuable therapeutically in collaboration with the theoretical grounding offered by the professional staff. Says O'Connell: "They [the paraprofessionals] are not set in the can't do's and this can be very therapeutic." Another professional staff member added to this theme by reporting: "They are spontaneous; they lack rigidity." Another stated: "Book knowledge can sometimes get in the way of feelings." Said another: "You have to work for two or three years in order to outgrow graduate school."

Some of the paraprofessional staff share common life experiences with clients due to similar ethnic and class backgrounds. Having staff members with backgrounds similar to the clients helps the clients feel more comfortable. This shared background is felt to be invaluable in formulating therapeutic strategies. In some circumstances the client is helped to "open up quicker, because sometimes titles [professional status] can get in the way," as one of the psychiatrists put it.

A major value of the paraprofessional, according to the center director, is that "they want to grow . . . they are hungry for something more, for self-development and training." This, he said, is very helpful in being effective with clients, because this need to strive provides a vital energy that translates itself into a greater attention to the clients.

A major theme which occurs very often in discussion with inpatient unit personnel is the way paraprofessionals and professionals complement each other. The center administration believes that the combination of paraprofessional plus professional staff has resulted in better care for the clients than if either professionals or paraprofessionals were employed exclusively. A statement from one of the psychiatrists sums up the attitude of the center toward paraprofessional staff: "I love them; I trust them and this increases as I work with them."

The attitude toward the use of paraprofessionals by the clients is reported to be generally good. Under certain circumstances, some clients are more comfortable with paraprofessionals than with professional therapists. The primary problems reported have to do with a worker's youth or hair length rather than educational background or competence. Occasionally people will be upset that they are working with a paraprofessional rather than a professional but complaints were reported in less than 5% of the cases. The staff reports that the majority of objections to working with paraprofessional staff come from two groups. These groups are older upper-middle-class women, and people from the lower economic class referred by social service agencies, who feel that they are being given second-class service unless they have the direct attention of the psychiatrist.

The paraprofessionals in the inpatient program perform many functions. As in most inpatient programs, the paraprofessional technician is responsible for the custodial needs of the client. This includes making certain that the clients remain on the ward, periodically checking on each client for whom they are the primary therapist. In addition, the technician helps to keep the ward clean, bathes clients when necessary, and helps the clients maintain their rooms, do their laundry, etc. The amount of time the paraprofessional technician spends in custodial care in comparison to more therapeutic contact will vary with the census of the unit. There are periods when almost all of the beds are occupied. The resulting demands on the staff members' time to care for patients' physical needs decreases the time available for structured therapeutic involvement.

In addition to the custodial tasks, the paraprofessionals in the Mid-Columbia Center have input on diagnosis and revision of diagnosis in cooperation with the psychiatrist in charge of the client. When a client is assigned to the primary therapists, they become responsible, as described earlier, for generating a treatment plan (SOAP chart) under the supervision of the psychiatrist. Once the treatment plan is decided upon, it is the primary therapists' responsibility to implement it. One aspect of this implementation is the charting of the progress of the treatment as well as evaluating effectiveness of the treatment strategies. The treatment plans will vary from client to client but will generally include the treatment modalities of individual and group therapy.

The paraprofessional primary therapist engages the client in a therapeutic relationship. Besides informal contact, the paraprofessional provides both one-to-one and group therapy either alone or with another professional or paraprofessional. The approach which is used is determined by the SOAP chart, directions from the psychiatrist, and the intuition of the primary therapist.

About half of the paraprofessional staff have studied and implemented specific therapeutic approaches which interest them. There is a center committee which meets to consider any innovation proposed by any of the staff, professional or paraprofessional. For example, a professional staff member who was interested in hypnosis was referred to study and work with a local expert to broaden his background before using it in the center. A paraprofessional specialist was sent to the Glasser Institute to study reality therapy. Among the kinds of innovations which the paraprofessional staff members have implemented are psychodrama, art therapy, expressive therapy[1] and music therapy.[2]

Selection and Recruitment

A great deal of attention goes into the selection of paraprofessional staff members. The center job description for the paraprofessional technician lists four important qualities that the person should possess.

Emotional maturity is the first quality listed. The job description describes as follows more specifically what is meant by maturity.

> [Maturity is] the ability to deal constructively with reality, the capacity to adapt to change, a relative freedom from anxieties, the capacity to find more satisfaction in giving than receiving, the capacity to relate to other people in a consistent manner with mutual satisfaction and helpfulness, the capacity to sublimate, to direct one's instinctive hostile energy into creative and constructive outlets, the capacity to love.

In addition, the job description emphasizes the importance of what is called the four "Rs":

- The *right* of an individual to intervene in another person's life
- The *responsibility* he must assume when he does intervene
- The *role* he plays in the process of helping
- The *realization* of his own resources

The next quality considered important is that of *communication*. Communication is defined as:

- Being able to direct or guide the therapist-client interaction to accomplish goals
- Being able to assess if communication is taking place, and to understand what, beside content, is being transmitted in the interpersonal process
- Having the ability to recognize when to speak and when to be silent

[1]Expressive therapy is an arts/crafts approach in which the client can play with clay, wood, pottery, etc.

[2]The music therapy group uses lyrics of popular music which are attractive to a client as a therapeutic device.

- Being able to wait and proceed at the client's pace
- Being able to evaluate

The next quality considered important is a high degree of *self-awareness*. The center wants the paraprofessional technician to be "aware of his own feelings and emotions (anger, pity, disgust, guilt, embarrassment, and sexuality) which may be aroused by clients during a counseling session."

The fourth general category of personal qualities in the job description includes such characteristics as *warmth, empathy,* and *genuineness*.

In addition to these general categories, specific traits are very important in the sort of person the center hires as a paraprofessional technician. These qualities are:

- Being self-motivated
- Being in good health
- Being able to tolerate ambiguity
- Being able to assess their own areas of weakness
- Being able to go to another for help
- Being open to learning
- Having no major bias, e.g., wanting to evangelize for a specific religion

Beyond these personal characteristics, the center is concerned with education and experience. They like to hire people with at least a bachelor's degree. The reason for this is not to require formal knowledge of the social sciences, but because it is felt that a college degree will provide personnel with the ability to read, write, and speak well. These abilities are considered to be very important.

The selection committee looks for applicants who have had experience in mental health service delivery. This experience is viewed as valuable both from the point of view of skills already learned and of indicating that applicants like the type of work. Volunteer as well as paid experience is considered useful in this regard.

The recruitment is done primarily through local employment agencies or newspapers. Applications are screened by a hiring team composed of the coordinator of the inpatient program, the head of the affirmative action committee, and four people who work in the unit. These four people are nurses and paraprofessionals.

After the initial screening, the remaining recruits are interviewed by the team. The inpatient coordinator makes the final decision with advice from the committee subject to the approval of the associate director for in-house services.

This same selection procedure occurs in all programs and on all levels. Thus, paraprofessional staff have input in the hiring of professional staff.

Training

Once hired, the new paraprofessional technician begins a three-month, three-phase orientation program. This orientation is primarily provided by the inpatient coordinator, mental health specialists, and other experienced staff. There is no specific time spent in any particular phase. After each phase is successfully completed, an evaluation report is written and the trainee moves on to the next phase.

In phase one, the new paraprofessional is oriented to the physical layout of the center and to the nature of services provided by the center as a whole. A detailed tour of the inpatient facility itself provides an understanding of the physical layout, and learning the location of supplies and equipment completes this phase.

In phase two, the new paraprofessional learns all the procedures of the inpatient unit including recordkeeping, admission/discharge procedures, diagnostic procedures, how to write a treatment plan, attending group therapy meetings, and witnessing one-to-one therapy.

In phase three, which generally occurs in the third month, the paraprofessional begins to assist in group and individual therapy. This is done by performing cotherapy with a paraprofessional mental health specialist or professional staff person who supervises the sessions and evaluates the paraprofessional's performance. The trainee then undertakes the task of being a primary therapist under the supervision of the rest of the primary therapist team and a paraprofessional mental health specialist. This task also includes aiding in the preparation of materials for staffing sessions.

After completing the three-month orientation procedure, the paraprofessional technician continues on-the-job training by working with and learning from those technicians and specialists who have had more experience.

The paraprofessional technician at this time begins in-service training which has three phases over a one year period. This in-service training occurs weekly in two-hour sessions, and is provided by professionals on the staff of the center, experts in the community, and paraprofessional staff with specific expertise. The training program is coordinated by a Ph.D. clinical psychologist who devotes half-time to its implementation.

The first phase deals with specific basic information and procedures in mental health service delivery. A few examples of the topics are: "Roles of Mental Health Technicians and Nurses"; "Commitment Law and Crisis Intervention"; "Management of Physically Assaultive Clients"; "Psychotropic Medications." This phase of the training occurs over about a six-month period.

The second phase deals with issues of self-awareness. Samples of the topics include: "Feelings of Self-Worth"; "The Client's Mourning Process"; "Effects of Therapists Concealing Their Own Needs"; and "The Implicit Threat of the Therapist's Self-Exploration."

The third phase of the in-service year focuses on an array of therapy models. The purpose is to develop in the paraprofessional technician an awareness and appreciation of different perspectives in approaching psychological problems. Three examples of this third phase are "Rogerian Client-Centered Therapy"; "The Gestalt Therapy of Fritz Perls"; and "Rational Emotive Therapy of Albert Ellis."

In addition to the two-hour weekly in-service training sessions, the center provides a specific recommended reading file of photocopied journal articles and excerpts from books which are specifically related to inpatient therapy needs. These materials are read and written comments are evaluated by the clinical psychologist in charge of the in-service training program. The center also has a general library which the staff is encouraged to use. Recently the center made arrangements to provide an in-house master's degree program in community psychology. This is done in cooperation with a nearby state university which grants the degree. The courses are taught at night at the center by center staff and by professors from the psychology department at the university. At present there are three paraprofessional staff members from the center enrolled in the program.

In addition to formal supervision sessions, the professionals on staff provide a great deal of consultation to the paraprofessional therapists and work with them in group and individual cotherapy formats. The paraprofessional therapists report that they feel very comfortable informally discussing difficulties they encounter in the therapeutic situation with the two psychiatrists, over coffee, lunch, or in free moments in the psychiatrists' schedules.

Supervision

The mental health specialists are supervised by the two Ph.D. clinical psychologists in a weekly ongoing supervision group in which cases are reported upon and evaluated by the professionals. In this supervision group any questions or problems in the mental health specialist's supervision task with the mental health technician are considered.

All the mental health specialists are paraprofessionals. They have the responsibility for the majority of the supervision of the technician's service delivery. This is done by direct observation of one-to-one sessions and cotherapy in group and individual sessions. Thus, monitoring and evaluation result in the further training of paraprofessional technicians.

Mobility

The upward mobility for a paraprofessional technician is a possibility but not a probability. According to the center director, only about 10% of the paraprofessional technicians can move upward. This problem is the greatest pitfall of the job reported by both the professional and paraprofessional staff. As one paraprofessional put it, "There is no place to go but out." The limits on the paraprofessionals' mobility does not seem to be their ability, but the lack of funds to pay them more as they gain experience and skill. The financial director put it very directly: "We train them beyond our ability to pay them." The center views the mental health technician position as a short-term one, about two years. The director sees the training received as being a means to a better job in another location.

However, the difficulty of upward mobility for the paraprofessional is compounded by the problem that experience gained in one center is not necessarily transferable. Therefore, the paraprofessional cannot move easily from a position of responsibility in one center to another, similar position elsewhere. One of the paraprofessional technicians interviewed had been in charge of two wards in a hospital in another state at twice the pay before she and her husband moved to the Richland area. While some paraprofessionals in the Mid-Columbia Center have found good jobs elsewhere because of their training, their lack of credentials causes transferability problems.

There is, however, some mobility within the center. Three mental health technicians have become mental health specialists. One former inpatient paraprofessional technician is now the coordinator of the outpatient program with administrative responsibility for many professional staff. The paraprofessional coordinator of emergency services is one of the three people in the catchment area who can authorize involuntary holds.

In summary, mobility at Mid-Columbia Mental Health Center is possible but difficult. Lack of mobility has resulted in the loss of a number of highly competent staff and sets up a pattern in which staff come on, are trained, gain skill, and leave for better jobs; then new staff must be hired and the cycle repeated. According to the director, "I have been concerned [with this cycle] for a long time and we've lost a lot of good people. The problem is money."

Status and Morale

The philosophy of a complementary team approach at the center contributes to the morale of the paraprofessional technician. The paraprofessionals report that they are respected, listened to, and appreciated. This, many said, is in sharp contrast to the treatment they had received in former positions in mental hospitals. As one staff member put it: "The administrator in a state hospital is God and beneath is a 'caste system.' But it's not like that here. Here they [the professional staff] know you, have coffee with you, know where you live. . . . It's a team! It always comes back to that."

The openness toward status and cooperation is carefully preserved. Says one professional staff member, "We have had psychiatrists who couldn't handle the openness. They 'came on' open and weren't, and it is they who are no longer here."

A paraprofessional technician describes the working relationship between professional and paraprofessional staff very well: "The structure is not rigid. Nobody peers over your shoulder. . . . If I need help I get it. The doctors are very informal; they will help you if you need it. They take what you say seriously. I matter!"

The morale among the paraprofessionals is excellent. The only two exceptions are the areas of salary and mobility. One paraprofessional staff member says, "If you are going to ask us to be good at what we do then you should have to pay us. It is not fair for the administrators to be able to sink roots and have the people helping people having to live like the Joad family in *The Grapes of Wrath.*" Another reports that he likes what he is doing very much and that the money is sufficient. However, he adds that if he ever wanted to get married and have a family he would have to find something else to do for a living.

There is a great sense of dedication to the center, to each other and to the clients among the staff. As one member put it, "We back each other up. We trust each other, we share our feelings, we care." When asked about his morale and why he chose the job, a paraprofessional replied, "It's watching a person bloom in front of you; I get chills talking about it. You watch them figure out their problems and come *alive.*"

When asked who set the tone for the feeling of openness and mutual trust at the center, the staff said that many people did but that Dr. Warren, one of the founders and current psychiatrist at the center, epitomized it. As one of the staff members expressed it, "He is an Albert Schweitzer of the desert. He seems to live by the adage of unconditional positive regard and I guess it rubs off."

Evaluation

The performance of the paraprofessional technician is evaluated periodically using a variety of means.

Informal evaluations occur on a daily basis. The mental health specialists evaluate performance based upon direct observation of the therapy sessions. The psychiatrists evaluate the technicians each time they report in a morning or afternoon staffing session. The clinical psychologists evaluate the technicians during in-service training.

There is a formal evaluation of service to clients done monthly by a utilization and review committee. This committee reviews a sample of the complete records of clients which are kept by the paraprofessional staff.

A formal in-depth evaluation of paraprofessional staff is carried out yearly after the series of three evaluations from the three-month orientation program. This evaluation is done by the coordinator of the inpatient program. It consists of a report form filled out by the inpatient coordinator and a self-evaluation form.

The evaluations of paraprofessional staff members show that their service to clients is very good and improves with experience. As a group, they are highly concerned with the clients they serve and want to continue to upgrade their skills to improve the quality of service. Those persons evaluating the paraprofessionals' performance were unanimously positive in their feelings about the paraprofessionals' capabilities in providing therapeutic care to the clients.

In Conclusion

Paraprofessionals play a vital role in the Mid-Columbia Mental Health Center. This is emphasized by the fact that 7 of the 20 programs are headed by paraprofessional staff. In the inpatient unit, direct service delivery is performed in the main by a primary therapist team composed of paraprofessionals working closely with professional staff. This collegial relationship, based upon mutual respect and trust, is a critical factor in the excellence of care provided. Because of the paraprofessionals' general lack of previous academic commitment to any specific theory of therapy, they are ideally suited to problem-centered treatment within an open ward and to new approaches to the care of clients.

Chapter 11

OUTPATIENT SERVICES

Introduction

Description of the Service Area

Outpatient services have been defined as an essential task of a community mental health center since the enactment of the original federal legislation that created funding for community mental health centers in 1963. National Institute of Mental Health guidelines presently consider that patients who need to spend relatively little time at the CMHC be provided appropriate outpatient treatment on a regularly scheduled basis with arrangements for nonscheduled visits during times of increased stress or crisis. The services provided should include diagnosis, evaluation, and treatment of psychiatric problems, and referral to other entities and agencies, as needed.

Although it is not necessary that outpatient services be available on a 24-hour basis, they must be available at appropriate times to meet the needs of the residents of the catchment area. Efforts should be taken to promote the accessibility of such service and to minimize unnecessary barriers such as waiting lists, restricted hours of operation, or hard to reach locations. CMHCs must also make outpatient care available during evening hours, weekends, at the patient's home, or at some other location when it is not possible for the patient to reach the center. Satellite clinics should be established when distances are too great or transportation inadequate for clients to reach the main office.

Selection of the Site Visited

Referrals received from regional Department of Health, Education, and Welfare offices, Washington, D.C. sources, and CMHC administrators were investigated. A final group of ten CMHCs were involved in the telephone survey for the selection of an effective program in the provision of outpatient services. The programs are scattered throughout the country in both rural and urban settings. The catchment populations served tend to be predominantly low-income and ethnic minorities. Every program operated out of at least one, and in some cases several, satellite clinics, following NIMH guidelines for availability and accessibility of services.

The centers surveyed made good use of paraprofessionals. Typically, at least 50% of the outpatient staffs were paraprofessionals and in some cases all direct services were provided by paraprofessionals with professionals providing supervision. The paraprofessionals can be used to provide more effective outpatient services in two ways. Since they are typically more economical to hire, they make it possible to extend services to a larger number of clients. The paraprofessionals' nontraditional orientation also broadens considerably the types of services offered by outpatient clinics.

There are two outpatient tasks which were provided exclusively by professional staff. Psychologists did all psychological testing of clients, and psychiatrists maintained full responsibility for client medication. Furthermore, long-term psychotherapy was generally considered to require the education and training that professionals have undergone.

All centers reported using paraprofessionals for in-clinic evaluation, diagnosis, one-to-one therapy and counseling, group work, family work, etc. In addition, centers described a variety of in-community work that was usually exclusively provided by paraprofessional staff members, including acting as advocates for clients dealing with welfare, employment, judicial, or other social systems; doing counseling in the client's home; consulting with community counseling programs; and training medical students to work in minority communities. The paraprofessionals, thus, supplement as well as complement the work of professional staff members.

Since its inception, the Orange County Department of Mental Health has shown a significant commitment to using paraprofessionals to provide effective and varied community mental health services. It is presently receiving funding through the Paraprofessional Manpower Division of NIMH, a continuation of New Careers funding begun in 1970.

The department has developed an extensive training program that involves paraprofessional and professional staff members in skills-based, academically accredited courses. New Careers funding was used, in part, to select indigenous ethnic minority persons from their community to undergo an intensive two-year training program that has resulted in their assuming responsible positions in the center. At present a similar effort is being undertaken with persons selected off of the county welfare rolls.

The department has developed a separate paraprofessional career ladder as a beginning toward solving the difficult problem of paraprofessional mobility. The mental health worker series contains four steps that can be attained with increased work experience.

The outpatient unit of the department's Region I office, the specific site visited for this chapter, makes use of paraprofessionals in order to accomplish a wide range of sophisticated tasks. They work in a peer relationship with professional staff members and share equal responsibility for all services delivered. The unit operates a satellite clinic in the city's minority community run entirely by paraprofessionals.

ORANGE COUNTY DEPARTMENT OF MENTAL HEALTH: A CASE STUDY OF OUTPATIENT SERVICES*

The Orange County Department of Mental Health (OCDMH) is a comprehensive community mental health program serving the 1.8 million people of Orange County, California. The present program is based on two major considerations in the delivery of mental health services to a large metropolitan population: the need for specialized services to meet special needs; and the need for readily accessible mental health services that are located close to the patients' homes. To implement these principles, the administration of OCDMH has developed an interesting organizational design. They have divided the county into six regional catchment areas. Each area has its own offices and a regional deputy director responsible for coordination of all services. From the central administrative headquarters, five special deputy directors maintain responsibility for the development of policy and assist the regional offices in the implementation of programs for the specific areas of Adult Direct Services; Children's Services; Alcoholism Services; Drug Abuse Services; and Training, Consultation, and Community Education Services.

*Contact: Orange County Department of Mental Health
2110 East First Street, Suite 109
Santa Ana, California   92705
714/834-6878
Attention: Frank Murillo, Service Chief
Adult Outpatient and Emergency Services
Mansell Pattison, Deputy Director
Training Division
714/834-3016

The OCDMH provides an excellent example of a mental health organization that makes substantial use of paraprofessionals in a wide variety of service areas. About one-half of the department's staff members are paraprofessional mental health workers; they range from indigenous community leaders with only a high school education to people with bachelor's and master's degrees. In certain areas, paraprofessionals provide up to 70% of the direct services. They perform approximately one quarter of all initial evaluations, individual counseling, and family counseling. They provide one-third of all group counseling services.

This chapter describes the outpatient services provided by the East Central (Region I) Regional Mental Health Office. This region, and particularly the outpatient unit, has a commitment to the significant, effective, and innovative use of paraprofessionals that is representative of the overall policy for the entire department. Paraprofessionals working with professionals in the outpatient unit share responsibility for all services that the unit provides to its clients. The sole exceptions are the medical responsibilities of the psychiatrists and the testing responsibilities of the psychologist.

By the nature of their experience, training, and formal education obtained while employed, as well as their broad service delivery responsibilities, the paraprofessionals are considered to be "professional" staff members of the center. All paraprofessionals are titled mental health workers, which is considered to be a professional occupational category. This chapter will maintain the distinction between paraprofessional and professional staff by referring to mental health workers—that is, those staff members who are not M.D.s, psychologists, social workers, or registered nurses—as paraprofessionals. Each paraprofessional staff member carries a full outpatient counseling caseload, runs therapy groups, does intake evaluations, and is involved in community work (indirect services). Most paraprofessionals also have an area of specialization that benefits a particular client population. Examples of these areas are gerontology, sex counseling, volunteer supervision, and couples communication. In addition, some of the paraprofessionals specialize in dealing with members of the Spanish-speaking community and the black community.

Background

In 1970, when OCDMH was first organized, there was no community mental health service system in Orange County. From the beginning, OCDMH was committed to an interdisciplinary organization that used new types of mental health personpower to provide a variety of direct and indirect services to the community. The department has grown from a small inpatient unit to a formal county department with 600 employees and a $27 million budget.

In 1970, three regional teams were created. Each consisted of one professional person with clerical support. Their primary function was to provide screening and evaluation services for county agencies. Rodney Chan, M.D., was the professional for Region I, and presently continues as the regional deputy director.

In 1971, under the auspices of the federally funded New Careers program, the department hired 16 paraprofessionals. This program was an effort by the National Institute of Mental Health's Paraprofessional Manpower and Training Division to incorporate the nonprofessional into the mental health delivery system. The purpose of this funding was threefold: to improve services to heretofore neglected populations; to develop career ladders for paraprofessionals; and to develop and implement an education and training system for the paraprofessional that provides for the attainment of college degrees, with credit given for life experience.

The 16 paraprofessionals lived in the local communities. They were all members of racial minorities, and were selected by community advisory boards. The paraprofessionals were hired for a two-year period into the trainee position of Mental Health Worker I. (Job mobility is discussed later in this chapter.) Half of the paraprofessionals' time was spent taking college courses or receiving training through the central training, education, and consultation division of the department. The other 50% of the time was spent working in the regional offices. All 16 trainees were placed in permanent full-time positions at the Mental Health Worker II level by the end of the two years.

Dr. Chan assumed responsibility for three of the new careerists as members of the Region I staff. They were an ex-Brown Beret, an ex-Black Panther Party member, and a woman who was and still is a major source of leadership in the local black community. These three people worked with the four professionals who by that time had also been hired as Region I staff members.

The relationship between the new careerists and Region I's professional staff was described as "strained" at first. However, a dialogue began between the two groups that resulted in the gradual development of a unified organizational team. The new careerists learned to work effectively within the system in order to achieve their goal of providing better mental health services to the people of their communities. These efforts resulted, for example, in the woman who was one of the original Regional I new careerists becoming coordinator of services for the regional outpatient satellite clinic. These paraprofessionals helped to educate the professional staff about minority cultural issues so that they were better able to serve minority clients. They also went into their communities and educated the people about the nature of the services available to them. In the words of the Outpatient Service Chief, Frank Murillo, "They were demystifying community mental health." As a result, minority population usage of the mental health services is greater than the minority representation in the area's population. Chicanos make up 22% of the population and 25% of the clientele seen in the regional office. Two percent of the population is black, while the regional office's clientele varies from 5 to 10% black.

In 1973, a second group of four trainees was selected for the NIMH New Careers program. This was the last time that persons were selected for a special training program until 1977. From 1974 to 1977, the department was flood-ed by applicants for paraprofessional mental health worker positions who had completed substantial college level work and, in addition, had clinically related experience. These persons often had M.A. degrees, and some even had Ph.D.s. Rather than use the New Careers funding for the selection and training of indigenous minority community paraprofessionals, the department hired paraprofessionals from this better educated pool. They then concentrated their training efforts on staff development at the regional level. This change in departmental New Careers selection and training strategy was described by a department administrator as due to the job situation in Orange County, which reflected economic conditions in the rest of the country at that time. In 1977, the department returned to its original New Careers strategy by selecting six persons from the county welfare rolls to undergo an intensive year of training as Mental Health Workers I in preparation for full-time positions in the regional offices.

The Adult Outpatient and Emergency Services Unit of Region I is the responsibility of Frank Murillo, M.S.W. He assumed this role two-and-a-half-years ago after a three-year commitment to the development of New Careers training as an employee of the training, consultation, and education depart-ment.

The present members of the Outpatient Services Unit include two psychi-atrists, one psychologist, four social workers, two registered nurses, seven mental health workers (paraprofessionals), and three clerical persons. They work out of a modern one-story building in the center of suburban Santa Ana. A satellite clinic is located about three miles away in the area's minority community. Some staff members rotate time between the regional offices and the satellite clinic, and others are full time.

Program Organization and Services

Operations.   Because the funds available for the delivery of outpa-tient services are limited considering the heavy demand for these services, Orange County (Region I) outpatient clients are seen primarily for short term therapy. Staff members describe the situation by noting: "Crisis work is our main concern. Our task is not to provide long-term psychotherapy. We try to teach people to become their own mental health worker; to help people to handle their problems. We take socially dysfunctional people and make them functional. This is different than helping people to pursue happiness through psychotherapy. Those cases we refer to professionals in private practice."

Some clients are chronic cases for whom medication and supportive therapy are indicated on a regular basis, but perhaps involving only one visit a month to the clinic. The psychiatrists are involved extensively in the medica-tion aspects of treatment, and carry only a small regular caseload. They depend on the judgment of the paraprofessional mental health workers, who act as primary therapists, to keep them informed about how well the medication is working, the presence of side effects, behavioral changes necessitating dosage modification, and other related problems. When interviewed, the professional staff members expressed full confidence in the mental health workers' ability to monitor these aspects of treatment and coordinate with the psychiatrists.

The individual therapy caseload averages about 25 ongoing cases for both professionals and paraprofessionals. It is somewhat less for staff members with larger responsibilities in other areas. Paraprofessionals determine the size of their individual caseloads. Cases usually are referred from the intake screening service. Each staff member does intake screening half a day a week with two staff members from other service areas (such as the day care service or inpatient service). If clients are judged to be suitable for outpatient therapy, then they become the responsibility of the outpatient staff member who participated in the intake session. This staff member either accepts the client into the ongoing caseload or seeks another therapist for the job. Suitability is informally decided on the basis of common knowledge of staff skills, abilities, and preferences.

A wide variety of therapeutic techniques is used by the paraprofessionals of the outpatient service. Techniques include gestalt therapy, crisis intervention, rational emotive therapy, and values clarification. Paraprofessionals learn appropriate techniques based on past experience, training sessions, and continuing education (see below). One paraprofessional stated: "A lot of my learning came from listening to how others handle similar problems."

Group therapy is commonly used and is considered an effective form of treatment. Each paraprofessional is a cotherapist in at least one ongoing group. Often patients are seen half a dozen times individually, and then are referred to a group for a longer period of treatment.

Most paraprofessionals go out in teams of two on emergency commitment cases involving the involuntary commitment of persons viewed as a danger to themselves or others. (Legally this action is covered under the California Penal Code 5150.) This type of work can be dangerous and causes much anxiety for participating staff members. It requires experience and an ability to be level-headed under stress. Only recently has the California law been modified to allow a mental health staff member other than a psychiatrist to certify persons for commitment under Code 5150. In the past, the paraprofessional mental health workers would do the job and use the signature of a physician to make it legal. Now mental health workers can make this recommendation on their own. All the mental health workers in Region I feel that it is only right that they be legally recognized as the responsible individuals.

Each client has a Problem Oriented Record (POR) written up by the primary therapist. This record indicates the nature of the problems, the plans for treatment, and the expected time for the plan. The POR is used by the therapist in organizing treatment sessions, and there are plans to use it as a peer evaluative mechanism. It is felt that the POR may help the clients to understand why they had to come for help. It also provides a written record so that continuity of treatment is maintained when, for example, a client moves from individual therapy to group treatment.

Use of Paraprofessionals

As noted above, Orange County has been committed to the use of paraprofessionals in community mental health centers since 1970. The outpatient and emergency services unit serves as a good model in this regard. Interviews at the site revealed several basic reasons for using paraprofessionals in this mode of service delivery.

Cost-effectiveness is an important reason for using paraprofessionals. The New Careers concept was developed, in part, to provide more services for the same funds; that is, to provide a more economical work force. In the state of California, funding provisions under the Short-Doyle legislation allow community mental health centers to bill for services provided by paraprofessionals at a cost identical to that of psychologists, social workers, and psychiatric nurses. Only psychiatrists bill at a higher rate. Private and third-party payers have shown a willingness to purchase equal services at equal prices whether or not the traditional educational degree is present. This equivalence of reimbursement combined with the lower salary requirements of paraprofessionals provides for more economical personnel.

Another consideration is the variety of life experience that paraprofessionals add to the typically homogeneous professional staff. The use of paraprofessionals with a heterogeneous mix of educational and experiential backgrounds can augment and enhance the traditionally structured and credentialed mental health employee model. Such an enrichment creates a staff better suited to service a variety of clients.

The minority paraprofessional staff members have made it possible for Region I to open and maintain the satellite outpatient clinic. This clinic, located in the minority community, is staffed entirely by paraprofessionals, and has greatly increased the accessibility of services for clients from this community.

Both the professional and paraprofessional staff members report that the unique abilities and experiential knowledge of the paraprofessionals are necessary to provide community oriented services. These are services that community mental health agencies are increasingly being required to supply. For example, consider the case of a family crisis in a poverty neighborhood. A personal understanding of the values and culture of that part of the community can prevent a mental health worker from making a serious blunder.

The paraprofessional often brings a special enthusiasm into the treatment of the very sick or chronic patient. A third of the present caseload in Region I is made up of the chronic/depressive type of client. Paraprofessionals will occasionally cause dramatic changes to occur, because they often do not believe in the hopeless prognosis of their clients, a prognosis that might discourage a professional. The center staff members believe in the notion of "health-engendering personalities" and that the success of treatment is related to therapist expectations. The selection of paraprofessionals is usually oriented toward this personality criterion, in contrast to the selection procedures for professionals, which typically are based on formal educational attainment.

In addition to individual therapy, group therapy, and intake screening, most paraprofessionals have responsibilities related to making the center work well. One mental health worker is in charge of volunteers. Volunteers provide a majority of the coverage of the outpatient service during the evening hours (5:00 to 9:00 p.m.). The volunteers are typically students in various college human service programs who are interested in obtaining experience with clients in an outpatient setting.

A mental health worker who is also the pastor of a church runs rap sessions for young people in the community, holds seminars at his church for couples, and gives talks on community mental health. Another mental health worker does program development consultation for a multipurpose service center that serves the Spanish-speaking community. A mental health worker who specializes in working with senior citizens is extremely active in the community. She is on various committees, such as the Orange County Council on Aging, which helps older people; she also works with a volunteer program, training people to visit and help senior citizens.

The service coordinator for the satellite clinic is a mental health worker. She is one of the original new careerists, and is a major political force in the black community. She is a member of various community boards, and her visibility gives credibility to the mental health center in the eyes of local residents. The paraprofessionals who operate the satellite clinic are also becoming recognized as a resource for information concerning the minority community. Recently, arrangements have been completed between Region I and the University of California at Irvine Medical School for the satellite clinic staff to provide consultation to medical interns. A broad knowledge of the minority community and the problems of its people is felt to be an important aspect of an intern's training, and a subject the clinic's paraprofessional staff members are well qualified to teach.

The administrative and professional staff regard the paraprofessionals as peers and there is no formal differentiation in job assignment (except medication and testing). However, it is interesting to note that even though the OCDMH has established a goal that all clinical staff should devote 20% of their time to indirect (community) services, paraprofessionals tend to spend more time than professionals in this activity. Community work involves a wide variety of tasks. In Region I's outpatient unit, each staff person develops skills and interests on an individual basis, with the assistance and guidance of Frank Murillo, who encourages his staff to work in the community. As cited above, these extra jobs include program development with a minority self-help agency, assisting a client to find a job, giving mental health talks to a school, etc. While all staff members describe such work as an important aspect of service delivery and essential to the success of the program, the professional staff generally have chosen to keep their in-community participation to a minimum and to emphasize clinical work at the regional offices.

The choice by professional staff members to adhere to the more traditional role requirements of an outpatient therapist does have a tendency to influence paraprofessional staff as role models. Possibly for this reason, some of the paraprofessionals are presently doing less in-community work than was accomplished in the past.

In addition to the influence of the professional role, the steady demand for therapy by clients works to decrease the time spent by paraprofessionals in the community. This demand is partially a result of the regional office's success in educating the community concerning the nature and usefulness of its direct services. Under these circumstances, when paraprofessionals allocate their time, they may tend to give priority to a more personalized type of help over community work.

Recruitment

Recruitment of paraprofessionals occurs at the county level. The county personnel department engages in fairly extensive advertising for each new position. Requests for individual positions originate at the regional offices. As described previously, the New Careers funding made selective recruitment of trainees possible, and a continuation of this funding, from the NIMH Division of Paraprofessional Manpower and Training, is once again being used for special recruitment and the ensuing training.

Selection

Frank Murillo, head of outpatient services, has full responsibility for staff selection. He bases his decisions primarily on the person's past experience in the field. The positions usually are directed toward a particular area of concern. For example, a mental health worker might be needed to work with clergymen in the community. To fill this role, the primary requirement would be experience working with the clergy. Ability to work with a particular ethnic group also is a typical requirement.

The backgrounds of the paraprofessionals providing services in the outpatient clinic vary considerably. The two poles of this continuum are extensive experience and involvement in community affairs, and experience in the provision of clinical services. To a certain extent, differences in paraprofessional background influence the manner of entering the system. Those paraprofessionals coming in as new careerists tend to be more community-oriented. The other paraprofessionals tend to have more clinical experience. Ideally, according to OCDMH administrators, a paraprofessional should combine both aspects of past preparation. It has been the practice of the department to provide supervision and training for the paraprofessional, with the intent of increasing awareness and abilities that may be lacking. Paraprofessionals are less resistant than professionals to learning about and working in the community. They do not have the professionals' well-developed awareness of traditional role definitions to impede their activities in this area.

Presently, aside from the New Careers effort, paraprofessionals are expected when first hired to have the necessary skills to accomplish their outpatient tasks. Most of the paraprofessionals interviewed reported extensive relevant experience. One had been a psychiatric technician in the Navy, then had worked in private inpatient hospitals, and finally had worked for the county in the methadone maintenance program. Another was a minister who was studying counseling; one was a social worker from India, who had traditional casework training but was unable to obtain certification in the U.S. without additional education here; one had been working for four years as a paraprofessional in the day treatment service; one had been a secretary for a university psychiatric facililty and, during her five and a half years there, had taken part in a wide variety of experiential training opportunities; and one had had four years experience working in inpatient services.

Training and Education

The major training responsibility is assumed by the Training, Consultation, and Community Education division of the central administrative offices of the OCDMH. This division has developed an extensive training program that provides skills training designed to be job-relevant, interdisciplinary, and interagency. The program operates on a quarterly basis that coincides with the schedule of the nearby University of California at Irvine. Approximately 15 to 20 courses are offered each quarter at the departmental administrative offices. The classes meet once a week for ten weeks, for a total of 30 hours. So far 75 courses have been developed. Each course has a title, course format, instructors, and an evaluation instrument. Ten of the department's 14 Mental Health Workers IV, the top of the paraprofessional ladder, work in the training, consultation, and education (C & E) division and teach courses. Line staff members from the various regional offices who have specific skills, including paraprofessionals, are also recruited to teach.

The courses are designed so that participants can gain skills in particular areas. Typical course titles are Rational-Emotive Psychotherapy, Gestalt Therapy Techniques, Treatment of Child Abuse, Consultation Procedures for School Counselors, Working with the Aging, Introduction to Group Counseling for Women, Helping Skills, and Behavior Modification Techniques. The training, consultation, and education division feels that it is entirely unnecessary to distinguish courses for a particular category of employee. Pretesting of personnel has shown that the need for skills is not related to the level of formal education. Any person from any agency or profession in the county may enroll if their work involves the skills and knowledge presented in a specific course. About one-third of the participants are from OCDMH and the other two-thirds are from over 30 different community agencies. This philosophy has provided a positive mix of interdisciplinary and interagency learning that has broken down traditional barriers and also promoted effective learning, sharing, and implementation of clinical tasks.

Various arrangements have been developed to establish certification and credit when courses are completed. Working agreements with the University of California, Irvine, and regional community colleges provide academic credits. Paraprofessionals can earn credit toward an A.A., B.A., or even M.A. degree. Completion of a course with a good attendance record and a passing grade on the final examination qualifies a student for a departmental certificate. These courses have achieved local recognition, and graduates find them a valuable addition to their personal resumes.

Each staff member has three hours per week allocated for career development. Consequently, a paraprofessional may participate in one three-unit college accredited course every ten weeks. Every paraprofessional from the Region I outpatient unit has taken a number of courses, some as many as eight or ten over a three to four year period. The New Careers trainees have made particularly good use of the educational arrangement afforded them. Of course, they had considerably more than three hours per week to devote to education during their two-year trainee period. At least half of these trainees, all of whom had a high school education or less, have obtained an A.A. degree within two years.

Supervision

Supervision and problem solving have developed into fairly informal processes. In the past, the formal meetings scheduled to accomplish these tasks were poorly attended and were, to quote a staff member, "more trouble than they were worth." The present informal system is based on the "professional" self-concept of the paraprofessionals, which implies that they do not need special supervisory mechanisms. These informal contacts are initiated by the staff members when they feel the need. Complementing this arrangement is the reported openness of staff intercommunications. Staff members feel they can talk to other staff members on an informal basis about problems or questions concerning the treatment of patients. They do not seem to have any fear of appearing ignorant. All staff members seem to make time available to accomplish this peer support and supervision.

Certain conditions are required if this informal supervision of staff members is to be successful. The past experience and level of responsibility of the paraprofessionals must be such that they know when to seek help. Problems can only be solved when there first exists the awareness that there is a problem. Access to a supervisor must be readily available whenever problems arise. Finally, mutual support among staff members requires generally positive and open intercommunication.

Mobility

In 1971, OCDMH developed a career ladder titled the Mental Health Worker Series to begin dealing with the problem of paraprofessional mobility. This four-step series is designed to promote upward mobility based on experience, and is reserved exclusively for paraprofessionals. A Mental Health Worker I trainee position requires only basic reading, writing, and speaking skills. This position is used for the New Careers trainees. The Mental Health Worker II position is the journeyman position, occupied by all paraprofessionals in Region I's outpatient clinic, as well as by the vast majority of the department's paraprofessionals. The salary range is $825–$1,102 per month. The requirements for the Mental Health Worker III or IV are progressively more on-the-job experience and/or formal education. These positions are reserved for paraprofessionals who are involved in administration and are occupied by 17% or 37 of the department's 217 paraprofessionals.

The paraprofessionals who function in clinical roles are still effectively limited to a single position—Mental Health Worker II. When interviewed, all staff members complained of this block to future job or salary movement. The typical paraprofessional staff member in Region I's Outpatient Unit has worked for the county for three or four years. They are very near or at the top of their rung on the career ladders and can see no further opportunity for financial advancement in the department. They enjoy the challenge and responsibility of their work, and generally feel that they could not find similarly rewarding occupations in another agency. They speak of returning to school to obtain an advanced professional degree, but most of these workers have families and could not take the time off.

The need for lateral mobility is a concern. The present job ladder can only be climbed by changing the nature of job responsibilities from clinical to administrative work. Paraprofessional staff members feel that a ladder should be created for advancement within the clinical field.

A frequent complaint related to job mobility is the salary differential between the paraprofessional and professionals. When staff members perform identical functions, the professional staff members are paid considerably more. This problem is recognized by both professionals and paraprofessionals.

Status and Morale

Apart from consideration of mobility and salary, the general tone of the outpatient staff is positive, with good relationships between professionals and paraprofessionals. In particular, the professionals are not threatened by the level of responsibility held by the paraprofessionals. The professionals feel they are working with people who can be trusted to do a professional job. They seek the assistance of paraprofessionals when they have clients who could benefit from a paraprofessional's particular expertise.

In Conclusion

The Orange County Department of Mental Health is clearly moving in the direction of defining the paraprofessional mental health worker as a professional in a way that differentiates them from volunteers, indigenous community workers, and aides or technical assistants.

Professionalism has been described in journal articles by the head of the department's training, consultation, and education division as consisting of: a commitment to a calling, with a service orientation; work that involves knowledge and skills based on specialized training or education; identification with peers in a formal organization; and autonomy in function restrained by responsibility. By comparing the mental health workers' present roles, particularly in the outpatient unit, against such ideas, it is evident that the professional nature of this work should be explicitly recognized.

Chapter 12

SCREENING SERVICES

INTRODUCTION

Description of the Service Area

Screening services provided by a community mental health center are of vital importance to courts and other public agencies that are attempting to determine the advisability of referring individuals to a state facility for inpatient treatment. These services are mandated by the 1975 Community Mental Health Center Amendments. The function of screening services is to reduce the number of inappropriate admissions to state institutions by providing valid treatment recommendations and by insuring that alternative, community-based treatment is available. For example, a judge may request screening services to help determine whether an offender is suicidal or otherwise seriously disabled and to determine the most appropriate location (given a "seriously disabled" diagnosis) for treatment as an alternative to incarceration.

In order to establish a screening service, program staff members should inform courts and other relevant public agencies of screening and treatment services available through the center. These services should include the assessment of the needs of clients, planning for the delivery of mental health and/or other needed services, linking of clients with the services identified, and provision of follow-up assessment of the progress being made by clients receiving treatment.

Selection of the Site Visited

It was difficult to locate screening programs that use paraprofessional staff members. This difficulty appeared to be related to two factors: (1) the relatively recent implementation of screening services and (2) the lack of credibility initially attributed by judges and other public officials to recommendations received from paraprofessional staff members. After surveying persons within both mental health and criminal justice disciplines, we received information on seven programs that might be suitable as models in this service area. Four of these programs are associated with community mental health centers.

The number of paraprofessionals in the screening programs varied widely, from 2 to 23. One important benefit gained by programs employing larger numbers of paraprofessionals is the capability of providing screening and/or intervention services for clients who potentially required care less comprehensive than inpatient treatment. Paraprofessional staff members are able to refer clients to a variety of community-based agencies, as well as to pay home visits to the clients and their families. As another example, they participate in making recommendations for offenders suspected of having drug- or alcohol-related problems.

The paraprofessionals are involved in various aspects of screening, including the interviewing of clients, the communication of recommendations to judges and other public officials, and the provision of counseling services to clients. The services that the paraprofessionals are least likely to perform involve the adminstration and interpretation of diagnostic tests and the communication of recommendations to public officials. Most of these paraprofessionals have B.A. or B.S. degrees. Since paraprofessionals with suitable training and experience in screening are very rare, the paraprofessionals in all the programs surveyed receive training as screening specialists from the professional staff members. The paraprofessionals are closely supervised by M.D.s or by other professional diagnostic specialists; any decisions for inpatient commitment are carefully reviewed by these supervising professionals.

The Roxbury Court Clinic was highly recommended by the Boston regional Department of Health, Education, and Welfare office. Located within a courthouse setting, the Court Clinic provides federally mandated screening services for adult offenders within cell blocks; it has the active cooperation of judges and probation officers. Supervised and trained paraprofessionals and professionals conduct extensive interviews of clients for whom inpatient treatment is being considered. Probation officers, arresting police officials, relatives of the defendant, and victims of crimes may be interviewed as part of the screening process. A psychiatrist thoroughly reviews each recommendation, and both he and a consulting psychologist are available to conduct in-depth diagnostic procedures. The clinic's staff members include a lawyer, a planning specialist, and professionals from several behavioral science disciplines. In addition to providing federally mandated services for adult offenders, the clinic provides screening services for clients for whom inpatient treatment is not under consideration. These clients include alcohol and drug abusers, and citizens whose mental health problems are associated with patterns of family violence. The clinic supplements screening services with therapy and social work services for adult offenders and for victims of crimes. In addition, federally funded drug and alcohol screening boards provide specialized screening services for clients being diagnosed for substance abuse; these boards maintain collaborative ties with community-based treatment agencies located outside of the mental health center.

Roxbury Court Clinic: A Case Study in Screening Services*

The Dr. Solomon Carter Fuller Community Mental Health Center is a state-owned and operated center giving comprehensive mental health and mental retardation services to a catchment area of 116,000 citizens (1970 census) in Boston, Massachusetts. It is under the auspices of the State Department of Mental Health. The Roxbury Court Clinic is a program of the Fuller Center, located in the Roxbury District Court, and affiliated with the Boston University Medical School. This chapter deals with the screening and related intervention and referral services provided by the Roxbury Court Clinic for adult defendants who have mental health problems.

The Roxbury court's jurisdictional area and the center's catchment area differ somewhat geographically, but the populations within the areas are nearly identical. Both areas include an inner city ghetto with large black and Hispanic minority populations. The unemployment rate within the court's jurisdictional area is about 40%, and only 15% of the residents have attended college. Each year about 10% of the residents of the Roxbury area appear before the court, although not all of these appearances result in legal action. The court deals with misdemeanors and lesser felonies and can imprison offenders up to a maximum of two and a half years.

The clinic provides some of the screening services now required by federal community mental health legislation. These services are provided for adult offenders, and the clinic's recommendations may influence the court to refer an offender to a state institution as an inpatient, or to an appropriate, less

*Contact: Roxbury Court Clinic
The Commonwealth of Massachusetts
Department of Mental Health
85 Warren Street
Roxbury, Massachusetts   02119
617/440-9500
Attention: Jacqueline L. Jenkins, Executive Director

restrictive treatment facility within the mental health center or community. The clinic actually goes beyond the federal requirements and the common practice of other mental health centers and both accepts and encourages referrals for clients suspected of having various types of mental health problems. Thus, whether or not the clients are viewed as having problems severe enough to require inpatient treatment, they are served by the clinic. In addition, the clinic offers therapy and social services both to defendants and to the victims of crimes.

With modifications, the clinic's approach could be transferred to a juvenile court. However, the clinic does not currently provide federally required screening services to juvenile courts or to the nonjudicial public agencies that occasionally ask for this assistance.

The clinic is notable for its collaboration with judges, probation officers, and community groups and for the complementary functions performed by the clinic paraprofessionals and by the professional staff members from several different disciplines. Paraprofessional staff members participate fully in all screening and intervention activities, with the exception of the administration and interpretation of tests. For example, paraprofessionals are as likely as professionals to be assigned as the primary screening agents for defendants against whom charges of murder, rape, and other serious offenses have been filed.

Background

The Fuller Center was established in 1969 with federal funding. All programs within the center, including the Roxbury Court Clinic, are under the jurisdiction of (1) an "area board," which is a community group comprised of residents of the catchment district; and (2) a board of trustees, whose membership is partially determined by the area board. The center employs paraprofessionals in a number of programs. Its staff members work closely with the area board.

The Roxbury Court Clinic was formed before the Fuller Center came into existence. Since 1956, many of the district courts within Massachusetts have had court clinics. The Roxbury Court Clinic, founded in 1960, differs from the other clinics in that it uses some paraprofessional staff members to provide a variety of services to clients and to establish ties with community-based treatment agencies. The clinic has dealt only with adult offenders since 1965, when jurisdiction over the juvenile population was removed by Massachusetts law from the Roxbury court.

In 1976, in a statewide move to consolidate a number of local mental health programs, the center assumed fiscal and administrative responsibility for the clinic, without making any changes in clinic operations. The center is planning to maintain the clinic operation in the courthouse, but will have its staff members participate as consultants in a centralized evaluation unit that will provide all the screening services required by federal law. The clinic staff will concentrate on cases where legal issues complicate the intake process.

Slightly more than 50% of the clinic's funds has been supplied by two special federal grants which finance two unique clinic programs. One grant, secured in 1973 from the Law Enforcement Assistance Administration, supports the clinic's drug screening board; the other grant, secured in 1974 from the National Institute of Alcohol Abuse and Alcoholism, supports an alcohol screening and referral program. The remaining funds are supplied by the state of Massachusetts Department of Mental Health through the Fuller Center budget. The federal funds are channeled through the state bureaucracy to Boston University, which acts as fiscal manager.

The clinic, in its present form, is the result of collaborative efforts by James Wells, the former executive director, and Judge Elwood S. McKenney, who has been chief justice of the Roxbury District Court since 1973. These efforts have been continued by Lester Bunyon, who became acting executive director in March 1977, when James Wells accepted a position as Assistant Commissioner of the Massachusetts Department of Youth Services.

The collaborative relationship between the clinic and the court reflects the mutual respect that has developed over several years. This respect developed in part because of active efforts by the clinic staff to establish ties with the court. Judge McKenney has said that because of these ties he feels that clinic staff members learned to appreciate the judges' insights. The judges and probation officers, in turn, began to accept the fact that screening and treatment services can be a useful aid to the judicial system.

In the beginning, the clinic staff members invited Judge McKenney to witness typical interviews in the screening process. The clinic staff cultivated relationships with probation officers by inviting them to participate in groups that refined and reviewed screening recommendations. As a result, Judge McKenney reorganized the probation department into four divisions (alcohol, drug, serious mental health problems, collection of moneys), three of which correspond with the screening services rendered by the clinic. He also required probation officers to work closely with the clinic staff.

Clinic referrals from the court have jumped three-fold since 1970. Previously, the clinic dealt mainly with traditional referrals for issues such as competency to stand trial; now it is given cases where serious criminal charges such as murder and armed robbery are combined with family and drug-related mental problems.

At present, the clinic employs 15 staff members, four of whom are full-time paraprofessionals and one of whom is half-time. Two of the paraprofessionals reside within the court's jurisdictional area; another was reared in Roxbury but now lives elsewhere.

The salary ranges and job classifications of staff members are as follows: M.D.: $31,100; Acting Executive Director (M.A. in social planning): $17,300; Social Workers (M.S.W.): $13,200–$14,200; Planning Specialist (M.A. in urban affairs): $5,200 (part-time); counselor and director of student training (M.A. in education): $8,500 (part-time); paraprofessionals: $10,600–$12,000. In addition, a part-time psychologist supplements the psychiatrist in providing the expertise required to diagnose complicated cases, while a part-time lawyer provides legal advice to the clinic. The total clinic budget during fiscal year 1976–77 was approximately $240,000. About $175,000 was paid during this period to regular and consulting professional staff. About $49,500 was paid to staff paraprofessionals.

Program Organization and Services

The Roxbury Court Clinic is located adjacent to the cell block where prisoners are incarcerated and within the courthouse building that includes the courtrooms, judges' chambers, and the probation department. The local police station is nearby. Clinic staff members can readily collaborate and confer with judges and with probation and police officers. Furthermore, the prisoners can easily be contacted or interviewed. The clinic includes a waiting room for clients, a large conference room, and a number of private offices for professional and paraprofessional staff members.

The clinic primarily screens clients referred by a judge, probation officer, or by themselves. However, anyone in the community can request and receive services. The clinic cannot ask to see clients. According to varying estimates, the clinic serves from 15 to 35% of the clients seen by the court. More than one-half of the screening services are rendered within the cell block. There are approximately 1,000 referrals annually; the clinic finds mental health problems in about 70% of these clients. The court accepts the clinic's treatment recommendation in about 90% of the 700 cases. The clinic cannot and does not wish to make recommendations for or against imprisonment, but the clinic recommendation can affect the trial date. For example, a trial may be delayed by a recommendation that a client be observed in an inpatient facility for 20 days to assess the client's competency to stand trial. The clinic can request a delay from the judge in order to complete a comprehensive set of screening procedures.

The clinic receives many referrals involving individuals who press charges as a way of obtaining social intervention services and/or help with mental health issues. These clients might not come to a mental health center, nor would they be served by a screening program that provides services only for clients possibly requiring inpatient treatment. A typical example is a wife who registers a complaint against her husband for assault. Episodes of family violence are frequent in Roxbury, and mental health conditions (e.g., alcoholism or the inability to communicate effectively) often contribute to the patterns of violence.

All clinic staff members are required to participate in screening activities and to set aside a portion of one day each week during which they screen defendants referred on short notice by the court. Not infrequently a judge will request an evaluation during a hearing in a courtroom; thus, quick service to the court is imperative. The paraprofessional or professional who conducts the initial interview becomes responsible for the client and, if appropriate, will arrange transportation to treatment facilities. In addition to the defendant, the clinic staff members may interview the victim of a violent crime, relatives of the defendant, the arresting police officer and the client's probation officer (if any). After all the relevant interviews are completed, the treatment recommendations for clients are reviewed by the clinic staff members in a case conference. The transportation to a state hospital is usually supplied by a court officer; in other cases the relevant treatment agencies usually supply the transportation.

A clinic paraprofessional staff member uses a monthly checklist to monitor the progress of clients referred to treatment agencies. The clinic staff have been concerned about the quality of service given by some treatment agencies for drug-abusing clients, but lack of funds has limited the clinic's follow-up activities.

For effective implementation of the clinic's approach to screening, both paraprofessionals and professionals require considerable training in diagnostic and interviewing skills. Professionals are not fully prepared for the clinic's screening activities, however, through traditional clinical training programs. Such traditional training requires supplementation by sociological information about crime, "street knowledge" provided by the community residents, and experience in the clinic's orientation program.

A court clinic has two clients—the defendant and the court. Staff members know it is a difficult and delicate job to serve both clients fairly. If a court uses a clinic to gather incriminating information on defendants, the clinic will soon lose its credibility in the community. The Roxbury District Court does not place the clinic in such compromising situations.

It should be noted that the defendants will often be highly cooperative with a clinic in order to receive treatment as an alternative to going to jail. For this reason, it is very important for a clinic to ensure that all the legal rights of its clients are respected. Thus, clients are informed prior to a screening interview that they may be asked incriminating questions. As another example, clients are told that they can reject the recommendations of a drug screening board.

In communications with the court, the Roxbury Clinic provides treatment-relevant information without providing evidence bearing on the charges leveled at the defendant. For example, the clinic might indicate that a marriage is "stormy" rather than saying that a husband admitted beating his wife. Thus, the clinic can make an appropriate treatment recommendation without revealing all of the facts to the court.

The clinic helps the judges to determine the reasons for commission of a given act, supplementing information provided by the traditional judicial process, and provides the judges with an alternative to the traditional options of incarceration, fines, and suspended sentences. The court, thus, is able to become a more humane institution by combining administration of justice with services designed to rehabilitate offenders and to enhance their mental health. Treatment, furthermore, can minimize the disruption of a defendant's mental health resulting from the family- and job-related consequences of incarceration.

All requests for screening are made by or through a judge on a form which requests an evaluation of a defendant's status in one of nine domains. Three of these categories correspond to the screening services required of mental health centers by federal legislation. They are: possible functional retardation; competence to stand trial; and danger to self or others. In each of these cases the judge wishes to know whether inpatient treatment may be appropriate for the defendant. Six categories are unique to Roxbury. The possibility of inpatient treatment is involved in two of these categories: drug dependency and alcohol abuse. The remaining four categories are: suitability for treatment at the clinic (as an outpatient); appropriateness of treatment as a condition of probation; evaluation for the presence of family-related mental health difficulties; and progress reports on clients who (1) have been receiving treatment services or (2) are nearing the end of a probation continuance period.

The clinic refers persons suspected of being mentally retarded to a screening service (Specialized Training and Advocacy Program) established by the Massachusetts Bar Association to help the courts. Once tested and interviewed, clients are referred to a treatment program appropriate to their disorder.

The staff psychiatrist is consulted by paraprofessional and professional staff members who have been assigned to screen clients for whom (1) competency for trial or (2) danger to self or others are being considered. These clients also frequently are tested by a consulting psychological assessment specialist. Staff members will also consult with the psychiatrist if they suspect that a client being screened for less serious conditions (e.g., alcohol abuse) may indeed be a candidate for inpatient commitment proceedings. Whenever possible, the cases of candidates for commitment are reviewed at the case conferences, which occur twice weekly for all treatment areas.

A consulting psychologist assists staff members who request case consultation. The psychologist deals with the clarification of treatment issues and suggests appropriate modes of intervention and/or remediation. The psychologist routinely conducts a one- to two-hour informal but structured interview with clients. The interview is designed to gather past and recent historical information; the session often results in clients' revealing significant precipitating factors. The psychologist often supplements the interviews with a selection of client-appropriate tests from the standard neuropsychological assessment and diagnostic battery, possibly supplemented by aptitude, achievement, or vocational achievement instruments. The selection can include any combination of the following tests: Wechsler Memory Scale, Bender-Gestalt Test,

Strong Vocational Inventory, Vineland Social Maturity Scale, Rorschach, Thematic Apperception Test, and the Minnesota Multiphasic Personality Inventory.

At that point, the psychologist writes and submits a recommendation to the staff member who requested the consultation. In the case of a civil or criminal proceeding, the report is forwarded to the judge who referred the defendant. The judge or the staff member requesting the consultation can review the report and recommend and request a session with the psychologist for explanatory information.

How does the actual screening take place? An example is provided by a cell block interview conducted by a paraprofessional staff member. As always in these interviews, the client was able to watch the clinic staff member take notes on a ledge-within-bars created for this purpose.

The client was arrested by a policeman for bothering a fifteen-year-old girl at a large ballpark during the weekend. The man did not actually harm the girl. When arrested, the man showed signs of extreme confusion. The client was referred by the judge for evaluation on grounds of possible danger to himself.

As a first step, the paraprofessional staff member established a relationship with the defendant. She asked him why he was arrested (he did not remember why) and showed him his arrest record to verify that she had the correct records. Next she explained the activities that had occurred in the courtroom. (The judge and attorneys often whisper during the court sessions, leaving the defendants confused and uninformed.) After explaining the clinic's purpose, she showed the client the evaluation request form and explained why the judge had requested evaluation for "danger to oneself."

Having established rapport, the paraprofessional asked the defendant about his activities during the past year. He described heavy weekend drinking bouts, his remaining sober during the week to keep his job, and his habit of having sexual relationships with prostitutes, rather than with his girlfriend, whom he "respected." When the paraprofessional asked about events prior to his arrest, the man claimed to recall nothing.

The paraprofessional staff member then consulted with the clinic psychiatrist, who diagnosed the man as having a problem with alcohol and as being a possible danger to himself. His defense lawyer was asked to go to his workplace to verify his good work record. (If a clinic staff member had gone, the defendant might have been fired.) Because the defendant had a good work record and no prior arrests, both the psychiatrist and staff members attending the case conference agreed to release the defendant on the condition that he would participate in an evening program at a community alcohol treatment center. (Placement in a halfway house might have caused him to lose his job, thus creating further mental problems.) The clinic requested progress reports from the alcohol treatment center, and the client was warned that the probation department would refer his case to the judge if he stopped treatment. Later, the client was scheduled to begin therapy with a male clinic therapist concerning his sexual relationships with women.

What characteristics make a treatment plan acceptable to a judge? An example is provided by a recommendation written by a paraprofessional staff member concerning a pregnant defendant diagnosed as being a heroin addict. The recommendation represented a consensus among members of the Drug Screening Board. WOMEN, Inc., is an inpatient treatment facility for female drug abusers with live-in facilities for their children. The collaboration between the probation officers and WOMEN, Inc., made it possible for the court clinic to make a recommendation acceptable to the judge.

> I find _____ to be a drug-abusing person in need of immediate medical attention. Although she displays a lack of motivation at this time, I feel she would take advantage of treatment as a means to ease the tension of the birth. Arrangements were made for _____ to enter Boston University Prenatal program where she would receive the sufficient medical care and also be involved with WOMEN, Inc., for the needed support and direction she desperately lacks. WOMEN, Inc., has agreed to accept her inpatient after the birth of the baby. The Drug Screening Board (DSB) office is willing to monitor this case with the help of close probationary supervision.

This recommendation is jargon-free, bears on the issues addressed in the screening request, and makes a realistic treatment recommendation. The judges are not concerned with complex diagnostic labels or the inner dynamics of personality problems; they do not appreciate recommendations that skirt the issues concerning the court and will not accept treatment plans that offer recommendations obviously insufficient for the problems at hand. In this instance, experience has shown that a recommendation for day care or for outpatient therapy would have been rejected by a judge as being unrealistic. For similar reasons, the clinic does not recommend treatment for drug pushers, because of the awareness that the judges wish to incarcerate convicted pushers. (Many times drug pushers are charged with felonies and their cases are transferred to the jurisdiction of the superior court.)

The Roxbury Court Clinic program incorporates a number of unique features. They include: clinic-based interventions for clients, drug and alcohol screening programs involving community-based agencies, procedures for screening retardates, planning of future programs, and training of graduate students.

Interventions.   The clinic provides outpatient therapy up to three times weekly on an individual, couple, or family basis for defendants, for relatives of defendants, and for the victims of crimes. Clinic therapists are able to deal with crime-related issues (about which most therapists are ill-informed) and to provide services in a neutral setting. Therapists, especially the paraprofessionals, may supplement office therapy with home visits and with social work activities.

Because participation in therapy sessions is often enforced by the probation department and ordered by the judge, not all offenders are internally motivated to receive treatment. On the other hand, these external factors can serve as an excuse for a client's seeing a therapist. Contrary to the custom in traditional psychotherapy, the clinic makes frequent efforts to persuade clients who have ceased participating to return for treatment. If these persuasive efforts are unsuccessful, the clients can be mandated to participate.

Because of its courthouse location, the clinic is able to provide or arrange treatment services to victims of crimes or to persons whose relatives have become defendants. The clinic may ask the court to suggest participation by victims or family members in relevant circumstances. In addition, a clinic staff member may write a letter to the potential client. These nondefendants tend to be battered wives, victims of statutory rape, or parents whose offspring are young adult offenders who have not yet left their parents' homes. Adult rape victims and children who have been abused by parents are referred to specialized treatment agencies.

In addition to the work at the clinic, one paraprofessional works almost exclusively on the streets and in homes. The following example demonstrates how the use of home visits (three times weekly), community contacts, and bilingual capability can assist clients.

A male client had been arrested for intent, while inebriated, to assault a resident in his apartment building. The screening process revealed that the man and his wife had been drinking and fighting and could not afford clothes or food. The paraprofessional's strategy was to reduce the couple's feelings of hopelessness by providing them with help. First he took the couple to a family service agency for counseling services and food. Next he took the couple to the Salvation Army and to a Catholic church center for money, food, and clothing. Then the paraprofessional smoothed over a family disturbance by visiting the client's sister. And finally, the paraprofessional wrote to the male client's mother in Puerto Rico to request money. (Previously, the mother had refused to send money, for fear that her son would drink with it.)

The Drug Screening Board.   Supported by a federal block grant from the Law Enforcement Assistance Administration (LEAA) to the city of Boston and hence to the clinic, this board consists of clinic staff members, paraprofessional representatives from eight community-based treatment agencies, and the probation officer in charge of the drug-alcohol probation unit. Originally (1971–1973), representatives from community agencies participated in the board without compensation. During 1973–1975, the grant supplied funds for paying community agencies for the consultation services of their program representatives. Now that funds are no longer available, the representatives again come to the clinic without compensation. About one-third of the clinic's clients are screened by this board. The representatives educate the clinic personnel about heroin and other hard drugs; in turn, the clinic exposure educates the representatives about diagnostic and treatment techniques.

The current coordinator of the Drug Screening Board is a paraprofessional. She is responsible for leading meetings, maintaining ties with the community agencies, and for coordinating follow-up checks, site visits, and other quality control procedures. It should be noted that the community-based agencies are reimbursed by third party payments for each treatment slot in their program filled by a client. For this reason, during Drug Screening Board meetings the representatives may occasionally compete for client referrals. Because of this fact, in Roxbury the coordinator of the board is an impartial clinic staff member with veto power over treatment recommendations of the board.

Prior to appearing before the board, each client is screened by a clinic staff member and then screened briefly by one of the treatment agency representatives. The board members discuss the evidence and then bring the client in for a group interview. This interview can be deliberately confrontational in style, so as to cause defendants to be truthful about their condition and to accept the fact that drug use is indeed a problem rather than a status symbol. The agency representatives, many of whom are ex-addicts, are especially wary and sensitive to the manipulative tactics that defendants may employ. Then the client is asked to leave the room while the board reaches a joint decision. Because the representatives are present, a treatment agency can make a commitment to accept a client. Then the client is brought back to hear the group's decision and to state his/her feelings about the decision. Clients recommended for clinic outpatient treatment may be required to come to the clinic two or three times a week for drug-detecting urine tests.

Alcohol Screening Program.   Supported by a federal grant from the National Institute of Alcohol Abuse and Alcoholism, this program maintains ties with representatives of 17 collaborating community-based treatment agencies. About one-third of the clinic's clients are found to have alcohol-related problems, including poly-drug abuse, although many of these clients are referred to the clinic for other reasons. The most common offense for alcoholic clients is a crime against a person, rather than against property. In the Roxbury community, alcoholism is more of a disgrace than drug addiction. The line between social drinking and problem drinking is not clear, because denial is one component of excessive alcohol use. Consequently, clinic staff members often need to conduct longer-term one-to-one assessments in a low-keyed fashion. Thus, the multiple-member screening format of the Drug Screening Board is not appropriate.

Screening for Mental Retardation.   The clinic maintains a collaborative relationship with Specialized Training and Advocacy Program (STAP), a state-funded screening and referral agency specializing in the problems of the mentally retarded. One of the program professionals acts as a liaison person with the STAP representative assigned to the clinic to screen clients suspected by a judge of being mentally retarded. The liaison person meets at the clinic with the STAP representative to discuss the disposition of cases and the progress of clients who have been referred by STAP to treatment programs.

Program Planning.   A part-time planning specialist helps the clinic staff members, including the paraprofessionals, to develop new programs, such as the alcohol screening program. Because the clinic staff workers are usually fully occupied by the daily demands of their jobs, the planning specialist provides the necessary objectivity and time commitment for gathering information, arranging meetings, and articulating alternative approaches. Her approach is to remain aloof from personnel and other day-to-day decisions in order to focus on the future.

Program Evaluation

Screening.   The screening services seem to be effective in providing appropriate treatment recommendations. Screening services, however, are only the first stage in the rehabilitation process. Their ultimate impact depends on the quality of services subsequently received by the clients from the clinic- and community-based intervention programs.

Clinic-based Interventions.   The clinic provides outpatient therapy services and community-based social services because these services would not otherwise be provided to the clinic's population. The efficacy of these intervention services (and of the screening services) is demonstrated by the fact that the five graduate schools in the area place graduate students in the clinic to learn intervention and screening skills. The clinic-based therapy services are limited, however, because clients often do not choose freely to participate and because 40 to 50% of clients drop out within the first month. (This dropout rate is typical for social service agencies.)

Drug and Alcohol Screening Programs.   These two programs have established successful collaborative relationships between the clinic and community-based treatment agencies. In addition, these two programs have significantly increased the awareness by judges and probation officers that alcoholism and drug abuse, while causing crime, are mental health problems for which treatment is appropriate. The programs also have educated the clinic staff members about the nature of alcoholism and drug abuse. Finally, the judges accept, at an 88% rate, the screening recommendations of the Drug Screening Board and of the clinic staff with regard to alcoholism problems.

The efficacy of the community-based drug and alcohol treatment program is less easily demonstrated. The clinic does not carry out thorough follow-up procedures. A sizable percentage of clients referred to the drug treatment agencies reappear at court. The community-based treatment programs probably vary considerably in the quality of services rendered.

Use of Paraprofessionals

The clinic staff members consider themselves and their colleagues to be professionals. A "professional" is defined by the staff members as a person who possesses the necessary skills, while a "paraprofessional" is a person who needs to acquire further skills for effective performance of the task at hand. (For the purposes of this chapter, however, the term paraprofessional will be used to designate persons with a B.A. degree or less.)

When the staff members were asked whether people without advanced degrees were necessary to the operation of the clinic, the members indicated that the clinic could operate no more effectively if the staff were comprised entirely of people with M.A. and higher degrees. One possible reason for this opinion is that most graduate training (with the exception of training to do diagnostic reports) does not prepare people for the duties of the clinic. Additionally, regardless of academic degree level, it would appear that to operate such a clinic, some of the staff members should be indigenous to the community and knowledgeable about its subcultures. The familiarity of the paraprofessionals with the Roxbury neighborhood makes them more knowledgeable than the clinic professionals about Roxbury community organizations and street life. This familiarity is also useful in communicating with the clients and in paying home visits. For similar reasons, many of the consultants to the Drug Screening Board from community-based agencies are ex-offenders who are able to provide input on the criminal subculture and on "games" that clients may play to manipulate clinic staff (although only one paraprofessional is an ex-offender). Thus the paraprofessional staff members in Roxbury allow the clinic to perform quality services at somewhat lower costs.

The paraprofessional staff members spend about one-half of their time in screening-related activities. Their remaining time is spent primarily in providing therapy and some social work services to clients. Because of their heavy caseloads, paraprofessionals tend to be underutilized by the clinic relative to professionals in home visits and community liaison work, areas in which paraprofessionals are particularly well qualified. Paraprofessionals do spend about 5 to 10% of their total work week in community public relations and consultation services.

All staff members, including paraprofessionals, are allowed to take on additional responsibilities based on their interests. For example, one paraprofessional is the coordinator of the Drug Screening Board and is also responsible for sending routine monthly follow-up questionnaires to agencies that receive referrals from the clinic. A second paraprofessional spends some time giving talks to organizations and carrying out liaison work with treatment agencies. A third paraprofessional pays home visits to clients and also observes the street culture and reports recent developments. A fourth paraprofessional consults on legal issues that arise in clinical cases. The fifth paraprofessional is involved in linking the court and the clinic and in follow-up of cases.

Recruitment

Paraprofessionals are not actively recruited; rather, they are hired from a pool of applicants or as the result of observation of their work-related competencies. Two of the paraprofessionals had sought and obtained secretarial jobs in the clinic setting. Showing an interest in and aptitude for clinical work, these secretaries were trained and promoted from within. Two other paraprofessionals are supported by federal revenue sharing funds provided by the Comprehensive Employment Training Act (CETA), and were hired as the most eligible candidates for the opening among those submitted by the city of Boston. The fifth paraprofessional, an indigenous Spanish-speaking male, was hired after the clinic had become acquainted with him through a community agency in which he was employed.

Selection

New positions are publicly advertised. Serious paraprofessional (and professional) contenders are then interviewed by a number of clinic staff members, including staff paraprofessionals.

The paraprofessionals are not required to have a B.A. degree or a mental health background. Two of the paraprofessionals hired had only high school diplomas at the time of employment. The clinic does not differentiate requirements for professional and paraprofessional staff members. Both groups are required to be at ease with the low-income and multiproblem population served by the clinic, and to be able, with appropriate training, to perform the required tasks under the high pressure circumstances not infrequently imposed by the demands of the court.

Training

The orientation period for new paraprofessionals requires six to eight weeks for completion, depending on the relevant experience of the worker. The new paraprofessional is oriented individually to the Roxbury system through a series of talks with the probation officers, the judges, and clinic colleagues, and by attendance at court hearings, case conferences, and the Drug Screening Board meetings. Screening skills are learned through a gradual shift from observing paraprofessional and professional colleagues, to conducting a screening session while being observed, to receiving intensive supervision while conducting screening by oneself, to screening without formal supervision.

The clinic administration arranges for some films and somewhat more frequently invites guest speakers to give talks or to lead discussions or training sessions on relevant topics. A more extensive in-service training program is currently being developed.

Supervision

Paraprofessionals receive one to two hours of one-to-one scheduled supervision weekly from the clinic professionals, focusing primarily on therapy cases; attention is routinely given to screening cases, however, when the paraprofessional is new at the job. Paraprofessionals rotate among supervisors to provide an opportunity for exposure to different viewpoints, and frequently consult informally with both paraprofessional and professional colleagues.

At the Roxbury Court Clinic, some staff members felt that both paraprofessional and professional workers involved in screening programs should be routinely supervised by professionals highly trained in diagnostic techniques and in the formulation of diagnosis-based treatment plans. For example, a supervising professional receiving a detailed psychosocial evaluation might suspect and subsequently detect the subtle cues of impending delirium tremens or of a condition of temporal lobe epilepsy that results in violent behavior when a client has been drinking heavily. These diagnoses drastically affect treatment plans. Supervision is especially important in cases where a client is being screened for commitment to an inpatient treatment facility. When any doubt arises in these cases in Roxbury, the psychiatrist does the complete screening procedure in collaboration with the relevant staff member.

According to the legal advisor to the clinic, if the paraprofessionals were not supervised by professional staff members, the paraprofessionals would not be covered by state laws protecting therapists from being forced to divulge privileged communications from clients. The Roxbury Court has not required clinic paraprofessionals to divulge communications from clients, but paraprofessionals in similar programs elsewhere may be subject to court orders requiring actions that conflict with the privacy of the therapist-client relationship.

Mobility

There is no job mobility for the paraprofessionals at Roxbury. Paraprofessionals cannot receive promotions except by earning a master's degree. At the same time, the paraprofessionals cannot find equally challenging mental health jobs elsewhere with equivalent or higher pay.

Three of the five paraprofessionals are enrolled in B.A. programs. Because of the heavy daytime demands of the court, these staff members attend evening classes. The paraprofessionals do not receive academic credit for their on-the-job learning experiences nor are they paid or given substantial time off from work to attend school.

Status and Morale

The paraprofessionals feel accepted as peers by the professional members of the clinic staff and report that competence rather than degree level is the basis for respect within the clinic. A new staff professional is oriented by the staff members possessing the relevant skills, whether paraprofessional or professional. Paraprofessionals and professionals receive the same quality and amount of supervision, represent the clinic on boards and through public speaking engagements, have private office space, and perform almost identical tasks.

The work is generally challenging to paraprofessionals. Because the clinic staff is small in number and occupies a compact space, numerous friendly informal contacts occur among the staff members. The paraprofessionals' salaries are supplemented by consultant assignments.

All of these factors contribute to high morale among the paraprofessional staff members. But the paraprofessionals are uniformly unhappy about receiving "less pay for the same work," the lack of job mobility, and being in temporary or, in one case, secretarial job slots. The paraprofessionals also do not feel that their job titles adequately reflect their competencies. Unfortunately, any changes in the base pay or in the job descriptions would require a change in Massachusetts state legislation, for the state controls the funds (with the exception of federal funds) used to operate the clinic.

The paraprofessionals do not experience problems related to their lack of advanced degrees with clients, judges, or with professionals or paraprofessionals from other treatment agencies. To these parties, paraprofessionals and professionals are all known as social workers. The judges do not differentiate between the recommendations and counsel from paraprofessionals and professionals. Other agency personnel readily accept the clinic paraprofessionals in consultation and liaison roles. Furthermore, the clients do not know or ask about the degree status of the counselors they see for screening or therapy services.

Some difficulties specific to the paraprofessionals do exist. Schools placing graduate student trainees in the clinic require that professionals provide the supervision. One professional did feel that paraprofessionals tended to be silent in planning sessions and thought they might see themselves as lacking adequate knowledge for discussing these issues.

Evaluation of Paraprofessionals

The clinic does not evaluate the performance of its individual staff members in any formal fashion. Accordingly, it is not possible to report statistical evidence about the effectiveness of the paraprofessionals, as a group or in comparison to the professionals. However, some anecdotal evidence bears on these issues.

Screening.   The screening services provided by the paraprofessionals seem to detect many clients who "do not belong in the criminal justice system." The clinic paraprofessionals appear to be able to recommend appropriate treatment services. The Chief Justice, the probation officer, the representatives from the collaborating community-based treatment agencies, and the planning specialist all reported satisfaction with the screening services performed by the paraprofessionals. In fact, the judges accept about the same percentage (90%) of treatment recommendations regardless of whether these recommendations are made by paraprofessionals or professionals.

Interventions.   No informal evidence suggests that paraprofessionals are less effective than professionals in rendering therapy services. The formal education of professionals, furthermore, does not prepare them to deal with this type of clientele. Home visits and the arrangement of social services from community agencies are probably carried out more effectively by persons familiar with the community or with its subculture. The clinic's paraprofessionals possess some advantage over the clinic professionals in this type of knowledge.

In Conclusion

The Roxbury Court Clinic provides screening and a number of subsequent intervention services at a critical period in clients' lives. By providing evaluations of defendants within the courthouse itself, the clinic is often able to divert persons with mental health problems from the penal system. Some of these clients require inpatient treatment. Other clients eventually receive day care or outpatient treatment for a range of less serious mental health problems. Clients with such problems are often not served by screening programs.

Paraprofessionals are a vital component of the operation of the clinic. They have proven to be capable of effective communication both with judges and defendants, and, under close professional supervision, they routinely perform psychological screening tasks. The use of paraprofessionals enables the Roxbury Court Clinic to make optimal use of its limited resources, as well as to employ staff members with an understanding of the unique problems of its clients.

Chapter 13

TRANSITIONAL CARE SERVICES

INTRODUCTION

Description of the Service Area

Community mental health centers must provide a program of transitional services for mentally ill catchment area residents who have either been discharged from a mental health facility or who would without such services require inpatient care in such a facility. Although closely related to follow-up care, a program of transitional services focuses on the need for adequate, sheltered community living arrangements. Such living arrangements are designed to foster a gradual, phased return to community living to the maximum extent possible for each person.

Transitional services may be provided in a variety of settings, including, for example, crisis hostels, foster homes, halfway houses, cooperative apartments, hotels, nursing homes, and boarding houses. The essential ingredients are appropriateness of the living arrangement to client needs, and provision of services to assist clients to recover from or overcome the handicapping affects of mental illness or disability.

The chapters on follow-up and partial hospitalization services contain descriptions of programs that overlap with transitional services. The interested reader may wish to refer to these two chapters for additional ideas on the use of paraprofessionals in a transitional services program.

Selection of the Site Visited

Attempts to locate effective programs in the areas of transitional services yielded a limited number of referrals. The relatively small number of referrals suggests the nationwide lack of development of programs using paraprofessionals in this service area.

The Weber Mental Health Center in Ogden, Utah, was recommended by the director of another Utah mental health center. In addition, the Denver Department of Health, Education, and Welfare regional office confirmed that the Weber Mental Health Center's Problems Anonymous Action Group (PAAG) program was a unique, effective community mental health effort that could serve as a model for transitional services.

Subsequent telephone calls to Ogden elicited a description of the paraprofessional program run for and by ex-alcoholics, ex-mental hospital patients, other paraprofessionals, and other persons living a heretofore marginal existence. The program had its beginnings as a self-help effort on the part of the inhabitants of Ogden's skid row, 25th Street. The administrators of the Weber Mental Health Center recognized in this incipient program the potential for providing care and habilitating many of the persons for whom they felt they were mandated to provide mental health services.

This combination of self-help and professional technical assistance has resulted in a program that is ideally suited as an effective model in the area of transitional services. Staff members provided detailed data on steadily decreasing state hospital admissions and police arrests for alcohol-related crimes in the locale. Laudatory reports from mental health investigators provided anecdotal confirmation. For example, Franklin Chu, coauthor of *The Madness Establishment,* recommended the project in a letter. He wrote: "The Weber County Center, in particular, impressed me with its range of alternatives to hospitalization and transitional facilities. For example, their sheltered workshops, where people make curtains on contract to condominiums, was a refreshing contrast to most occupational therapy programs."

PAAG, INC. (WEBER MENTAL HEALTH CENTER): A CASE STUDY IN TRANSITIONAL SERVICES*

Nestled in the foothills of the towering Rocky Mountains, just east of the great Salt Lake, is the city of Ogden, Utah. From this location, the Weber Mental

*Contact: Weber Mental Health Center
      350 Healy Street
      Ogden, Utah   84401
      801/399-8391
      Attention: Rhett Potter, Center Director
            Kirby Potter, Program Administrator,
               Direct Services

Health Center (WMHC) provides services to 140,000 residents of Weber and Morgan counties.

This chapter will describe the services provided by Weber Mental Health Center in conjunction with one of its components, known as the Problems Anonymous Action Group (PAAG, Inc., pronounced "page"). These services are included in the center's organizational design under the heading of direct services and they have no other formal identification. However, the activities that are undertaken include all of those that federal guidelines, as described by the National Institute of Mental Health, specify should be provided as transitional services by a community mental health center.

PAAG is a private, nonprofit corporation, staffed entirely by paraprofessionals, offering a wide variety of community outreach and sheltered living services. The majority of PAAG consumers are long-term alcoholics or ex-state mental hospital patients.

WMHC, in addition to PAAG, is organized into five teams. The teams are: Intake Services, Legal Services, Ethnic Services, Youth Services, and Direct Services. Direct Services include crisis intervention, outpatient, inpatient, and partial hospitalization. The head of Direct Services, Kirby Potter, M.S.W., is responsible for managing WMHC's unique relationship with PAAG.

Legally, WMHC and PAAG are separate entities. Although staff members from the center played an essential role in the founding and growth of PAAG, it was deliberately split off from WMHC. This was, in part, to give its staff members credibility with the street clientele who might be resistant to traditional mental health workers. This legal arrangement provides a number of additional benefits that will be described later in this chapter. Presently, PAAG operates much as a satellite center to WMHC. WMHC is the funding source for PAAG, "a wholly owned subsidiary." Their relationship is made formal through a contract between the two organizations. This contract specifies the mental health services that PAAG will provide for the center.

PAAG is operated by volunteer members with the supervision and assistance of paraprofessional and professional employees from WMHC. Together they offer important services to a heretofore neglected and needy population. A hotel for the skid row alcoholic provides a place to sleep, to eat, and to receive encouragement to make a better life. Sheltered living situations provide communal housing and rehabilitative programs for ex-state mental hospital patients. A street drop-in center provides several important services: a place for coffee and conversation, immediate medical attention, and referrals to appropriate agencies. An extensive court diversion program helps to interrupt the cycle of repeated incarceration that is typical of skid row inhabitants.

These activities and others will be described. The paraprofessionals who are responsible for PAAG's daily program depend upon the professional staff of WMHC for support, supervision, training, and problem-solving assistance. The center depends upon the paraprofessionals to do a job that WMHC feels is necessary, mandated by their funding sources, and "what we simply could not do alone" according to the clinical director.

Background

In the latter 1960s, Rhett Potter, M.S.W., and C. Wallace Dalley, M.D., both employed by the state hospital in Utah, began to consider the idea that mental health care could be effectively delivered in a community setting. Concerned citizens in Utah were also examining alternatives to the incarceration of mental patients. The two men advanced their notion to a colleague, Douglas C. Conrow. This nucleus of three began to lay the groundwork for a community mental health center.

Rhett Potter began organizing the center in 1968. The ideas leading to the center were not widely accepted in the mental health field, and this led to difficulties in the design and funding of the program. The theory that guides staff members at WMHC regards mental health problems in a different light from that of the traditional medical model. At WMHC people are not treated for "mental illness." Rather, clients are thought of as individuals who have difficulty in functioning in one or many areas of living. The person's difficulties cause him/her to behave in ways that are unacceptable to society. Mental health services are seen as a way of identifying and modifying unacceptable behavior in a community setting with community feedback. "Mental illness" is not seen as disease requiring removal from the community.

WMHC's definition of mental problems requires an innovative approach to treating troubled individuals so they can learn to live in the community and to satisfy such desires as the need for self-esteem, close personal relationships, and family ties. The mental health consumer is approached as part of the community and given the help to remain there and to develop a more successful life-style.

The philosophy is based on the premise that people learn abnormal behavior, and, like any learned behavior, it can be unlearned. Because clients are not labeled mentally ill, Weber Mental Health Center workers do not attempt to cure anyone, but try to change or modify unacceptable behavior. Says Dr. Dalley, "We believe that some people are out of phase with society and exhibit unacceptable behavior."

On January 5, 1970, Weber Mental Health Center opened its doors. Opening the center was not a simple set of tasks, and keeping the doors open has required an intensive commitment by its staff members. Nevertheless, by tenaciously holding to its direction, WMHC has become a unique model of community mental health services.

WMHC is housed in a modern brick and steel building in Ogden. This building contains the center's administrative offices, conference rooms, data operation, and staff members' office space. However, very little client service is given in this facility. The WMHC teams do most of their work in community facilities such as schools, churches, neighborhood centers, outreach centers, in the homes of clients, and on the street. In addition to these outreach settings, WMHC also has developed close working relationships with other human service agencies (such as law enforcement agencies, the courts, legal services, social agencies, youth agencies, probation, family services, and the schools), and it provides services directly to these agencies. By using existing community resources and working cooperatively with other agencies, WMHC can deliver services throughout both Weber and Morgan counties.

History of PAAG Inc.   PAAG is a private, nonprofit corporation chartered by the Utah Secretary of State to raise funds and provide services for its membership. Since no profits accrue, PAAG has members rather than stockholders. All full members are, or have been, consumers of the mental health services. The PAAG Creed states:

> The Problems Anonymous Action Group is devoted to advancing human dignity by providing a meaningful involvement for people on the fringe of society. This goal is based on the assumption that all individuals regardless of their race, color, creed, sex, or previous history have one or more areas of competence which can be used for the good of society and the improvement of the individual. Our role is to change weaknesses to strengths and support abilities until each individual becomes a solid member of the PAAG subculture, a culture whose norms and values are congruent with the larger society and yet still personally rewarding.
>
> The PAAG philosophy unequivocally rejects labeling individuals and rejects the incarceration of people with noncriminal behavioral problems. Any behavior may be normal or abnormal depending on its social context. This view furthers the dignity and personal liberty of the individual and fosters responsibility in the community.
>
> It is the conviction of PAAG that this creed will be vindicated by time, and this philosophy shall endure.

PAAG came into being in September 1970, when a handful of people who lived in the 25th Street skid row area of Ogden, Utah, formalized their informal alliance, calling themselves the "Problems Anonymous & Alcoholic Group." All of the original members were consumers of mental health services in one way or another. They were state mental hospital patients, mental health center clients, alcoholics, and others who are often viewed by social service agencies as isolated from the rest of society. The life-style on downtown Ogden's 25th Street—known as Two Bit Street—provided community rather than isolation; the Two Bit Street people felt that they had much to give to each other, although the more affluent members of Ogden society looked upon them with disapproval. They had a vision that their shared way of life could become the basis of a mutually supportive organization, and the name they chose for their new association reflected its anticipated membership.

From the outset, PAAG has been a cooperative self-help venture. The earliest activities engaged in by the original association of 25th Street people included very basic social activities such as "coffee and conversation," get-togethers at members' hotel rooms, dances, and Friday night movies. PAAG members cleaned up movie theaters and a dance pavilion in exchange for free passes to movies and dances. It is important to note that these activities were initiated by people who would be viewed by traditional mental health standards as dependent personalities.

Meanwhile, Rhett Potter at the Weber Mental Health Center became aware of the activities of the 25th Street people and recognized the potential value of the group as an extension of the center's programs. Potter felt that WMHC could realistically offer only outpatient and crisis intervention services to the 25th Street residents. On the other hand, he realized the usefulness of coordinating and complementing these services with socialization and recreation activities, which could only be handled outside the structure of WMHC. Accordingly, discussions were held between the WMHC staff and the PAAG leadership that resulted in a partnership. PAAG, as a nonprofit entity, would provide social and recreational opportunities to the 25th Street community, while the Center would provide direct mental health services as well as other needed logistic support.

Over 200 chronic alcoholics inhabit Ogden's Two Bit Street. These people were the first concern of PAAG and a target for outreach planning by the WMHC. After PAAG members and center staff made a trip to Albuquerque in late September 1970, to visit an innovative, flexible alcoholism program, PAAG established a "skid row" coffeehouse to provide alcoholics with an alternative to wandering the streets, retreating to their rooms with a jug, or sitting out time in jail in the local drunk tanks. The Salvation Army provided the space as well as a pool table, while WMHC provided coffee, tobacco, and telephone services. Originally open six hours per day, five days per week, the coffeehouse soon was running seven 12-hour days a week in order to accommodate the demand.

The experience gained in operating the coffeehouse convinced both PAAG and WMHC that a cooperative effort by a mental health center and its consumers could significantly affect the quality and usefulness of the services rendered to community residents and that it required substantially less capital to operate than a more traditional unilateral approach. Accordingly, WMHC and PAAG began to expand their vision of joint service delivery. Consideration was given to the possibility of incorporating PAAG as a nonprofit organization, which would allow PAAG to assume a legitimate place in the mental health structure as a subcontractor, and would also allow PAAG much more freedom in developing direct service programs and facilities for community residents.

At an organizational meeting held one wintry night in December 1970, 50 members of PAAG decided to incorporate under the name of "Problems

Anonymous Action Group," thus maintaining the PAAG acronym. The board of directors for the new corporation came out of the PAAG membership present at the time of incorporation. Rhett Potter and the WMHC staff assisted PAAG in writing a constitution and bylaws, and the articles of incorporation were filed; the corporation undertook its new mission immediately.

Both PAAG and WMHC agreed that residential facilities were sorely needed for alcoholics and mental patients. Until such sheltered living arrangements could be provided to consumers, any further program development would be hindered. It was also clear that because of the regulations and guidelines imposed on WMHC by the funding sources—such as the requirement that there be established ratios between the number of staff members to residents, or that state codes for nursing homes be followed—resident programs would be extremely expensive and beyond the scope of the WMHC. PAAG, as a separate and distinct organization, was in an excellent position to develop and operate such sheltered living residences at a much reduced cost.

The corporation's first venture into the realm of residential facilities, appropriately christened PAAG I, resulted in a boardinghouse for women. WMHC assisted PAAG with money and advice. In essence, PAAG generated the idea of a boardinghouse for women, and WMHC provided most of the political and organizational expertise necessary to create the facility. PAAG took responsibility for operating and maintaining the boardinghouse, while the funds necessary to operate the residence were provided jointly by the residents (from their employment income, public assistance, and other forms of income) and by the WMHC. The WMHC also provided a paraprofessional liaison team to handle problems of service delivery to the members of PAAG, and to encourage PAAG members to learn strategies for program decision-making.

The first residents of the boardinghouse were four women who were inpatients at the center. Two were members of PAAG as well, and all four had local or state hospital inpatient experiences. It was felt that, while these women could no longer benefit from the medically oriented inpatient program, they could profit from a group living situation.

The corporation's next accomplishment was the development of a men's residence hotel in a 10-unit apartment building. The interior of this building was completely cleaned, painted, and refurbished by PAAG members prior to its opening. All of the labor necessary to meet building code and health requirements was done by persons who, until this time, had a history of dependency on social agencies. At this point, the men's residence was designated as PAAG I, while the women's boardinghouse became PAAG II.

PAAG has not been uniformly successful in its ventures, nor has its evolution been without obstacles. In its six-year history, PAAG has opened and closed several facilities and programs. Some of these changes were related to the growth of PAAG; however, others were due to false starts and insufficient planning. Growing pains were also felt in the development of the board of directors. The Two Bit Street people had little experience with the middle class concept of board meetings. Responsibility for regular attendance, as well as the responsibility for organizational decision-making, was not easily shouldered or understood. Within the board, a core of committed individuals provided continuity and singleness of purpose, while a number of other directors failed to accept responsibility for more than a short period of time. When PAAG first came into existence, biweekly board meetings were scheduled, and it was often necessary for a WMHC liaison person to round up each of the board members for the meeting. Since then, however, a transformation has occurred for most PAAG board members, and the staff members at WMHC perceive this change as a tremendous success and growth for PAAG.

PAAG does its work with two primary target groups within Ogden. One group, those individuals with chronic mental problems, is found throughout the two-county catchment area. The other group, those persons with severe alcoholism problems, is located in one specific section of town, the 25th Street skid row area.

Twenty-fifth Street is a society in miniature. The district covers some 10 square blocks of downtown Ogden, bordered by the railroad yards on the west, city hall on the east, and extends one block to the north and south along 25th Street. The area is typical of the run-down inner section of a small city. Several hotels are located here, surrounded by taverns, pawnshops, "greasy spoon" cafes, vacant lots, and abandoned small businesses. The street is a society within, but separate from, the districts that surround it. It is the area where largely forgotten people continue to cope with their living needs in a marginally successful manner.

The street scene is not an easy life. As in any local community or district, there are rules to the game of living there, and the rules of 25th Street are comparatively severe. An alcohol or money debt owed, a favor that is due, or simply some disagreement is oftentimes a matter of life or death. Physical danger and brutality are frequent on the street. Even when these conflicts are absent, the life-style of a skid row alcoholic is far from the relative security and safety accepted as the normal situation by the rest of the community. Physically the 25th Street residents bear the scars of past fights and the evidence of slow degradation of the body from continuing use of alcohol.

Uke's Cafe has been the gossip center and hangout for the local alcoholics for many years. Located in the heart of 25th Street, it is operated by Mary Nakaishi and her husband, Yukio. Mary, who has been written up in a *Time* magazine article as the "Angel of Twenty-fifth Street," is a rare individual who takes care of virtually anyone who passes through her life. She provides street information (such as the immediate whereabouts of a particular resident, who is in trouble with whom, and the like), helps new arrivals find a place to stay, makes sure the "regulars" are okay if they do not show up at the cafe according to their usual patterns, serves food (she has a credit system with many customers), and operates as general counsel to street residents.

It is only by taking advantage of what might be termed the natural resources of this impoverished area, such as Mary Nakaishi, that WMHC and PAAG are able to operate successfully. Mary's important involvement served as an inspiration in the formation of PAAG. She is still actively involved in street life and is a continuing source of assistance to PAAG and the center. Mary's position on 25th Street is unquestioned, both by the residents and the mental health workers. She was essential in obtaining community support in establishing PAAG.

By taking the time and the energy to learn how the 25th Street community operates, WMHC began to see how the center could affect the unfulfilled needs of the residents. This knowledge did not come easily. When the mental health staff members first became visible along 25th Street, many local residents did not trust them. Residents felt that the mental health people posed a threat in undercutting the existing rules of the street, so the first paraprofessionals were recruited from the 25th Street residents. Their initial role was as bodyguards for the professionals from WMHC. The knowledge, or street savvy, of these paraprofessionals was invaluable in assisting the planning and needs assessment phase of the venture. In developing a working relationship with some of the street residents, WMHC sowed the seeds for a different kind of service delivery system, one which eventually resulted in PAAG, Inc.

Jack Clark, a 25th Street resident who was one of the first people to work with the WMHC staff members providing protective services, became a prime motivator in the organization of PAAG, and directed its first programs. After the basic PAAG structure had been developed, Jack Clark was murdered in one of the many altercations that regularly occur on the street. Clark's absence is still heavily felt at the center and among PAAG members, even though he has been dead several years. To them he symbolizes the productive *and* difficult path traveled by PAAG in gaining access to the 25th Street community.

Program Organization and Services

Transitional services are divided into four basic units organized around the current programs of PAAG, Inc. The Alcohol Diversion Program deals with the chronic alcoholic, providing nursing services and problem solving for the transient population in and around the PAAG hotel. PAAG I is a men's residence hotel for the homeless inhabitants of the area, operated by four paraprofessionals. The Sheltered Living and Day Care Program component has responsibility for the chronic ex-state hospital patients living in the PAAG II residence, as well as for a boardinghouse and five local nursing homes. This program also offers services to PAAG members in a day activity center where long-term mental patients learn basic living skills. The Socialization Team is composed entirely of PAAG members serving as volunteers who organize a broad range of activities in the community.

Alcohol Diversion Program.   The primary responsibilities of this program—also referred to as the 25th Street Unit—are nursing and crisis intervention. Unit workers operate along 25th Street and provide direct medical care to those on the street, as well as help in making living arrangements, assistance in locating and obtaining financial resources and meals, a sympathetic ear for problems, and appropriate counseling. The unit is made up of three paraprofessionals and one licensed practical nurse. The nurse provides first aid and physical examinations and dispenses medication. One member of the unit works directly in the jail and with the courts to divert alcoholics into available human service programs outside of the criminal justice system. Once diverted, contact is maintained with the individual, and the unit makes every effort to keep him or her out of jail. The unit also staffs the alcoholic day contact center, which offers a program for local alcoholics who are not residents of PAAG I. Here, street people can congregate for conversation, coffee, and PAAG activities and find a unit staff member to listen to a problem. The licensed practical nurse works out of the contact center.

PAAG I.   When the building housing the men's residence hotel was purchased by PAAG, it was completely run down. Through a series of negotiations, agreement was reached with the local health and building inspection officials so that PAAG could refurbish the building, and, with the exception of the electrical work, all renovation was done entirely by the residents of the hotel. Located on Wall Street, just off 25th Street and across from the railroad yards, the hotel can house 22 men. There is a kitchen and meals are provided. A recreation room, a meeting room, and individual bedrooms for the residents make up the rest of the building.

The day at the hotel begins at 7:00 a.m. Residents are expected to get up, dress themselves, and clean their rooms. The men then go downstairs to the dining room for breakfast. Following the meal, the men are encouraged to do something—work around the hotel, work at an outside job, go out on the street, play pool at the hotel, watch television, or just have a conversation. In the late afternoon, the residents return for a meal. After dinner, residents may sit around talking, or go out. Everyone is expected to be back at the hotel by 10:00 p.m.

The philosophy of the hotel is simple. Those who choose to make use of its facilities must follow the daily structure. This, in turn, establishes a regular and healthy pattern in the men's daily behavior. The men receive encouragement and advice from the paraprofessionals who run the hotel and who act as role models—continually showing residents that a change in their lives can take place. They are not made to feel guilty or turned away if they go out on a binge. The guiding principle is: "If they want to get drunk, they should do it elsewhere. If they want to change, we'll help them!" A resident who returns to the hotel in an inebriated state is asked to remain in his room until he sobers up. If he does not do this, but makes a nuisance of himself instead, he is asked to leave.

The Sheltered Living and Day Care Program.   PAAG II is a residential home for women who typically have a history of mental problems; it can house nine women. In addition, the Sheltered Living and Day Care Program is responsible for a boardinghouse and five nursing homes which are contracted by WMHC to provide room, board, and care for other PAAG members.

The Day Care Program is offered to these residents, none of whom has lived as an independent person for some time. The paraprofessional staff members teach such basic living skills as learning to tie shoes, to dress, and to use eating utensils, as well as the proper care of furnishings and the basic equipment of a home. The residents also learn communication skills. A model apartment is located at the sheltered work facility to allow residents to experience a living space that they control and to teach individuals what is required to live alone. The program includes specific subjects, usually taught by the staff and visiting instructors, such as courses on sewing, manual arts, music, civics, crafts, and on many other topics.

Actual contract work is done by the members of the sheltered work programs, such as janitorial services and envelope stuffing and mailing. All earnings from such contracts are paid directly to the workers involved. In addition, program members decide on activities to pursue outside the sheltered work facility. These activities, which include sightseeing and trips to museums, libraries, and parks, are intended to encourage active involvement in community and social activities. The program is sheltered, but continually encourages individuals to assume greater responsibility for their living situations.

The Socialization Team.   This unit is composed entirely of volunteer PAAG members who organize a broad range of social activities for the rest of the membership, including residents of PAAG I and II. Many PAAG people lack ongoing relationships. The Socialization Team, however, is able to generate ongoing activities, such as periodic parties, movies, dances, group music, holiday dinners, and outings that allow all members social experiences and encourage continued relationships.

Program Staffing.   There are presently 10 paraprofessionals and the licensed practical nurse working in transitional services programs. They can be divided roughly into three groups on the basis of funding. In practice, there is considerable overlap and cooperation in terms of task performance. PAAG I, the hotel, has four employees; the Alcohol Diversion Program has four; and the Sheltered Living and Day Care Program has three. Salaries range from $6,020 for a mental health worker to $15,000 for the paraprofessional executive director of PAAG. Kirby Potter is the only professional staff member with direct involvement in PAAG programs. Rhett Potter, the Center Director, and C. Wallace Dalley, M.D., the Clinical Director, maintain responsibility for broader pilosophical and organizational matters.

At present (Spring 1977) there are only two females among the 11 employees. One of these staff members is the nurse; the other woman is a paraprofessional worker in the Day Care Program. It was felt that a woman staff member would not be appropriate in the men's hotel. In the other programs, although women were recruited, very few applied for the positions. Racial minorities compose one-quarter of the staff.

Program Evaluation.   Although the PAAG I program is relatively small in terms of numbers, it has had a significant effect on street activity. This can best be illustrated by the reduction in total yearly public intoxication bookings in Weber County Jail. In 1969 there were 2,505 arrests for public intoxication; in 1970, 2,530 arrests; in 1971, 2,623 arrests. In late November of 1971 the PAAG I residence hotel was opened. However, it was not until mid-December that it was in full operation and filled to capacity. In 1972 the total number of bookings for intoxication dropped to 1,993; in 1973 the number dropped to 1,608. Some 1,500 arrests were made in 1974. In comparing jail records of individuals before and after involvement with PAAG programs, the PAAG I resident achieves a greater than 50% reduction in arrest and jail time.

The PAAG program provides medical services on the street. The licensed practical nurse from the Alcohol Diversion Program makes hundreds of yearly street contacts. If the alcoholics served had gone to the hospital emergency room, the cost to the taxpayers would have been approximately $25.00 per contact. The cost of providing this medical care is significantly less expensive because it is taken care of in the community.

Sixty-seven clients were supervised by the Sheltered Living and Day Care Program during 1972. State hospital statistics for 27 of these clients show that these individuals represented over 100 years of prior state hospitalization. During 1972 the entire group of 67 persons required only 18 days of hospitalization. It is felt that the main reason for this success in the reduction of hospitalization was their achievement of a stable position in the PAAG community.

During 1972, 13 clients lived in PAAG II. Collectively they represented over 47 years of prior state hospitalization. The cost of providing services to this group while at PAAG II was $10,567. Had they spent the same amount of time at the state hospital, it would have cost $85,932.

In the last six years of operation (since 1970) all state hospital patients who have participated in PAAG have been returned to the community. In this time only two readmissions have occurred. The remainder of these persons have been maintained in their community without major incident. Clearly, the operations of PAAG have had a dramatic impact on its two biggest populations.

The Socialization Team component is a major facet of the PAAG program and is made up entirely of PAAG members working as volunteers. The input from PAAG staff comes primarily in terms of referrals. Each week referrals are made to the PAAG board regarding who may be included in the social activities. The board and PAAG citizens also provide names of individuals who may gain by participating.

During 1972 over 225 different individuals attended PAAG social activities, and over 1,000 social contacts were made. In 1974 the total number of contacts increased to more than 4,000. These social activities included a weekly arts and crafts class, a bingo night, bowling night, Friday outings, weekly coffee and conversation groups, a cribbage and pinochle night, Saturday socials, and special events (Christmas, Thanksgiving, award banquet, and the like).

Another measure of the success of PAAG operations comes from Quarterly Benefit Reports that are developed for all WMHC programs. The purpose of these reports is to understand program delivery in terms of the program's action and its impact on the service community. The entire process is monitored to increase knowledge and understanding of working program models. A sample problem statement, taken from the second quarter report for 1976, follows:

> PROBLEM: In Weber County there are many people whose social isolation and resultant inappropriate behavior constitute a very noticeable mental health problem. This is particularly prevalent among the 100 center clients who fit into the area of chronic clients and also those 200 plus individuals who live in Ogden's 25th Street area.
>
> OBJECTIVE: Adequate revenue from PAAG I and from PAAG II will be generated. Improvements will be made in PAAG I to insure continued approval by the City Health Inspector, Building Inspector, and Fire Marshal. All social functions will continue to be maintained by PAAG Incorporated and it will be given responsibility for at least 50% of the finance generating work activities designed for clients.
>
> a.   Maintain at least 65% paid occupancy in PAAG I during 1976.
>
> Paid occupancy for the first half was 163%. (Percentage based on financial data. A contract with the federal prison system created the financial prosperity.) This objective was met for the first half.
>
> b.   Maintain at least 75% paid occupancy in PAAG II during 1976.
>
> Paid occupancy for the first half was 96%. This objective was met for the first half.
>
> c.   Maintain a minimum of 2,500 contacts with PAAG people during 1976.
>
> During the first half of 1976 the total number of contacts was 1,924. This objective was met for the first half.

    d.   Maintain active PAAG membership of at least 150 people during 1976.

PAAG membership of 180 people was maintained. This objective was met for the first half.

METHOD: 1. Jim Pelton (the paraprofessional director of PAAG) will be responsible for collecting rent for all residents of PAAG I and Cary Stark (the supervisor of the sheltered living program) will be responsible for collecting rent for all residents of PAAG II. 2. A contract will be entered into between the Mental Health Center and PAAG, Inc., requiring PAAG to supply at least 2,500 contacts with chronic clients during 1976.

EVALUATION: Kirby Potter (head of WMHC Direct Services) will be responsible for monitoring the methods on a quarterly basis. The objectives will be evaluated on the basis of the material gathered by the Data Component of the Agency on a quarterly basis.

WMHC operates PAAG programs on a budget that is presently $245,000. Federal funding for the alcohol and day care programs directly contributes $112,400. Revenues from the men's hotel contribute $44,000. The additional $88,600 necessary for PAAG program operations comes out of the Mental Health Center's general fund.

Use of Paraprofessionals

The use of paraprofessionals is an integral part of the transitional services delivered by WMHC. Professional staff members at WMHC rely heavily on paraprofessionals to accomplish the tasks involved in rehabilitative, recreational, supportive, and sheltered living services. WMHC uses paraprofessionals because their salaries are less and because they have intimate knowledge of the community, flexibility of approach, potential for training in the center's philosophical model, ability to be role models for clients, and desire to engage in community outreach work. It must be remembered that the establishment of PAAG was a cooperative venture between the mental health center and community people. Alone, probably neither partner would have been successful. The autonomy and self-help nature of the PAAG programs are therefore dependent upon recruitment of many staff members from the ranks of those being helped.

    WMHC provides services in the area of transitional care, using three types of workers: the professional staff from WMHC, the paraprofessionals, and the volunteer membership of PAAG. The three groups work together with a common goal in mind—to increase the potential of their clientele for functioning with relative autonomy in their chosen community.

Each type of worker offers to the cooperative effort a unique combination of a life experience and formal training. The amount of formal training experience decreases from professional to paraprofessional to volunteer. Conversely, the amount of applicable life experience is at a maximum with the 25th Street volunteers and is typically minimal among the professionals. These two types of experience are viewed in Ogden as necessary and complementary to each other.

The members of PAAG, particularly those who volunteer their time and energy to the various tasks, have a commitment that is solely theirs. Their lives are being affected and improved. They actively participate in this change. This is not only representative of a "good value" but is becoming increasingly recognized as a major criterion for truly effective social or individual change, i.e., people doing for themselves.

Presently, one-third of the paraprofessionals have been recruited from the ranks of the active PAAG members. These are people who, had PAAG not been created, might well have lived out relatively useless lives. They have combined an intimate knowledge of their community and a set of individual talents, skills, and desires, with the training and encouragement of the WMHC professionals. This set of circumstances has allowed them to be of major benefit to the people of their community.

Recruitment

Often employees begin their involvement in PAAG programs on a nonpaid basis. There is much opportunity for volunteer commitment. Volunteers are usually ex-consumers of the mental health services, but they can also be college students wanting to participate in a meaningful community activity.

Whenever possible, persons with direct knowledge and experience in the system are recruited for employment. This occurrence is not infrequent or tokenism; it happens with regularity. Jim Pelton, the current director of PAAG, serves to illustrate the point. He was in Ogden one day when his car ran out of gas. He immediately went on a three-month drinking binge and ended up with no money and only the clothes on his back. This binge drinking was a typical, almost lifelong pattern for Jim. He was one of the original members of PAAG. Gradually he became more involved with WMHC on a volunteer basis. Still later, Jim became the manager of the PAAG I hotel. For the last couple of years he has been the executive director of PAAG.

The varied histories of the paraprofessional staff point to possibilities other than volunteer work as background to future employment. Government programs such as the Job Corps or CETA have provided the money to hire people. Two of the paraprofessionals worked out so well on this basis that when their government funding ran out, the center provided the money to hire them full time. Two others had worked as paraprofessionals at the state hospital. Their experience, reported reliability, and positive attitudes facilitated their recommendation. Their desire to engage in more meaningful work in the community was an important consideration in their being hired.

Selection

The selection of staff members at WMHC has evolved from the center's experiences in the community, from carefully following the development of programs, and from following guidelines imposed by Weber County personnel. Sometimes the needs of the community, the program, and the county are not the same. WMHC's role is to balance these considerations in the selection of staff.

Several key features are evident in the staff selection procedures at WMHC. The center began with community input and a community orientation. The ability to deliver direct services and maintain community relations remains, to this day, a primary consideration in the hiring policy. Other considerations are to match the experience of a worker to the service requirements of the role, and to look for a strong commitment to the objectives of WMHC.

The head of Direct Services, Kirby Potter, M.S.W., maintains full responsibility for all hiring. He works closely with his paraprofessional staff members and solicits their opinions on personnel selection. For example, recently the hotel needed a night shift staff person. Two of the paraprofessionals joined Mr. Potter while he interviewed an applicant. They asked only a few questions. Afterwards, the three discussed the applicant Mr. Potter was in favor of hiring. One of the paraprofessionals said he didn't think it would be a good idea; the other supplied the reason. The applicant had been on duty at an Alcoholics Anonymous program that past winter. One of the 25th Street inhabitants came into the building out of the cold and had a bottle with him. Instead of simply asking for the bottle, the applicant yanked it from the man and hit him over the head with it. This and similar acts had earned the applicant a street reputation that would be detrimental to the PAAG program. Needless to say, the man was not hired.

Training

Kirby Potter is responsible for training at the center. Almost all personnel undergo a rigorous 12-week training program. Both professionals and paraprofessionals undergo identical training experiences. This is a general orientation to the helping field, to casework, and to the center philosophy. Textbooks, case studies, lectures, role playing, and the like constitute the course materials. Weekly quizzes and final examinations are given, and grades are distributed.

A second phase of training consists of field experience. New personnel are paired with experienced workers in the areas in which they need to have involvement. They are paired with several different workers in order to provide them with diverse experiences and to share the training responsibilities.

Supervision

Supervision is primarily the responsibility of the paraprofessional supervisors of the three programs. Kirby Potter is available as a problem solver, but the supervisors handle the day-to-day responsibilities of their individual programs. The paraprofessional supervisors have gained this trust on the basis of their past work experience.

The nature of the work of the PAAG programs requires that paraprofessional employees exercise a great deal of individual responsibility, flexibility, and creativity. Most work happens on the street and requires an ability to make immediate decisions that are sound.

Mobility

There is limited mobility in PAAG programs for paraprofessional staff because the present positions have been filled for a long time by the same employees. The four persons employed at PAAG I have been on the job for an average of three to four years in a program that is only six years old. The executive director of PAAG, who began as a volunteer in 1968, is an example of the past job mobility of paraprofessionals. Since all employees are paraprofessionals, it is probable that future supervisory positions such as the executive director's will be filled from present workers. CETA and Job Corps personnel have also gone on to become full-time, paid employees.

PAAG employees have different feelings about their future as paraprofessionals. These differences usually relate to their past experiences. Those employees who started as PAAG consumers may have found in PAAG the first meaningful, socially acceptable experience in their lives. Their role provides such satisfaction to them that to move on to a different organization is inconceivable. Some of the other employees see PAAG programs as less of a career. They value what they are doing, enjoy the people they work with, but see the limitations of the job, in regards to salary in particular, as too big a factor in their own lives. The paraprofessional staff members occasionally leave their positions to work in a much less satisfying job at better pay.

Education

Educational opportunities for paraprofessionals are excellent. The center believes that furthering the formal education of its paraprofessionals provides for better work performance. This is seen as occurring in two ways. Knowledge from the content of the courses can be applied to the tasks of service delivery, and the experience of dealing with a formal educational organization can be carried over to working with social service and judicial bureaucracies.

One paraprofessional came to WMHC with just a year of college. While he was employed, he received his B.A. from Weber State College and then his M.S.W. from Utah State University. He has gone on to become the Director of the Utah Department of Aging. Another paraprofessional is just now receiving his nursing degree.

The center is committed to paraprofessional education by offering tangible help to staff members. It varies from case to case, but includes up to 50% paid time off, with the Center paying for all tuition, fees and books, arranging work schedules around school requirements, and creating half-time positions.

Status and Morale

PAAG workers have a self-image of their role as individuals who are important helpers in the community. The workers feel they are crucial to the goals of PAAG and have very positive feelings about their status. Morale is not a problem. In general, the workers feel that their activities are an essential part of the treatment process and that this role is recognized by the professionals at the mental health center.

The primary concern of PAAG workers at present revolves around inadequate pay. Currently all the workers feel that the pay is low or that they are being underpaid for the work they perform. One worker suggested that PAAG employees should have a pay scale more equivalent to that of the professional employees of WMHC.

All paraprofessionals expressed positive feelings for their professional director, Kirby Potter. His—and the center's—resources for keeping the programs functioning smoothly were continually acknowledged.

Evaluation

All Direct Services staff members are evaluated on a monthly basis. Kirby Potter has devised a point system to compare performance with salary levels. Performance is rated in four weighted categories. The category titled *office requirements,* which includes such variables as "time put in at job," "attendance at meetings," as well as other similar measures of basic performance, is weighted 10%. *Paperwork,* which includes "quality of case notes," "quality of social histories," "necessary monitoring forms filled out," and the like, is weighted 15%. *Activity,* such as "number of clients seen in individual counseling," "caseload size," "time spent in outreach activities," "number of people supervised," and "number of groups held," is weighted 30%. *Output measures,* such as "number of terminations," "recidivism of caseload," and "length of stay of inpatient caseload," are weighted 45%. Points are assigned for each variable. The weighted sum is then compared with the average point total for all personnel. This comparison is matched with a comparison of the individual's salary relative to the average point total for all personnel. Finally, this comparison is matched with a comparison of the individual's salary relative to the average employee salary. Thus, an individual might be performing 25% better than the average employee. If his salary is below the average, and if this trend continued for the year, then he would merit a raise. An interesting feature of the reliability of this measure is a good correlation with Kirby Potter's knowledge of his staff, both in terms of their work and their personal lives. He stated that his confidence in the numbers was due to the accuracy of their reflection of his subjective viewpoint.

In Conclusion

A fundamental lesson that the PAAG programs teach is the existence of latent abilities, skills, talents, and the like in all persons. By helping people to help themselves, Weber Mental Health Center has achieved significantly broader mental health services provision than is accomplished by proponents of a traditional illness and cure model. Thus, for anyone interested in beginning a similar kind of program, the first step would be to search for self-help groups with which to begin a relationship.

The potential benefits of a separate nonprofit corporate entity such as PAAG, Inc., should not be overlooked. This arrangement provided not only financial benefits to the implementation of programs in Ogden, but also allowed the center to gradually relinquish more and more responsibility to the PAAG board of directors as their organizational skills increased with experience.

Working in a skid row area to provide mental health services can be a dangerous undertaking. Three lessons were learned by WMHC to minimize, to some extent, the risks involved. The first is to establish rapport with key inhabitants of the area, realize that their knowledge of the culture of their community is necessarily extensive and useful. Their judgment on decisions should be considered at all times. Second, be aware that mental health movements will be perceived as a threat by established petty criminals who flourish in these domains. They have to be dealt with. One way of accomplishing this in Ogden was to repeatedly communicate to them a lack of interest by the center in their activities. Finally, the population to be provided services will be leery of "mental health." In Ogden, the PAAG employees are called PAAG workers, not mental health workers; their salaries come through PAAG, Inc., not the center; they are indigenous to the community, not outsiders; and the philosophy that they learn to guide them involves much more than just mental health concepts.

Chapter 14

TRENDS ACROSS PROGRAMS

The programs we visited differed in many respects, including size, geographic location, ethnic composition, and philosophy. Yet, in the course of gathering information for the case studies in this book, we noticed a number of common themes and common features. Although we had not planned a formal study of the common characteristics of these programs, we feel that the observations that follow in this chapter point out certain areas of program functioning and structure that are important in the development of effective programs.

Further, research on organizational health and success supports many of our observations and conclusions. And, since the use of paraprofessionals in CMHCs is a relatively new phenomenon, we would like to suggest some general policies which might serve as guidelines for similar programs.

Program Planning

In all but one of the programs studied, substantial planning was done prior to the beginning of the program. In several cases planning grants specifically financed such activities. The center directors were involved in the planning of the programs in 10 of the 12 cases. In five programs the planning was done almost entirely by mental health professionals. Community people participated very actively in the planning in six of the programs, and where community planning predated involvement by salaried staff, community boards have tended to maintain considerable authority.

In programs where planning was carried out only by professionals, this phase of program development took less time than planning efforts which involved the community. However, interviewees in community-planned programs felt that the extra time and effort associated with community involvement was very worthwhile because it generated continuing community support and valuable input in the planning process. Community involvement seems particularly important in programs where close ties with the community and other agencies (e.g., drugs, alcohol, aftercare) are critical. Program staff emphasized the need, when necessary, to actively recruit community involvement before beginning a program. One center director actually returned federal funds rather than start a program without full community support. In two cases, mental health staff held planning meetings with community representatives in bars or restaurants because some of the community people felt more at ease in such settings than in the mental health offices. At one center, mental health staff personally transported community members from their homes in order to ensure attendance at the initial meetings. Such extraordinary efforts are often necessary and important in making programs fit the needs of the community and in making the community receptive to the programs.

An active board of directors can assist in ongoing planning by questioning program priorities, suggesting policies, and serving as a bridge to the community at large. The great majority of the programs we studied were served by boards of directors who were highly involved and showed a continued interest in them.

Those programs which were site visited tended to devote resources to planning as an ongoing part of program operations long after the initial planning phase was completed. While hard data about ongoing program planning were not gathered as a part of the present study, the "self reports" of these effective programs indicate more planning than most centers we have visited in other capacities. This supports evidence about the relation between planning and program effectiveness found in a previous statistical study (Blanton & Alley, 1977) in which the continued use of a technique of program development planning and evaluation was significantly related to ratings of program success.

Short-term program planning and decision making in general tended to involve a high proportion or even all of the staff. Regular meetings of all staff provided an ongoing assessment of program operations which served as a basis for future planning and also enhanced intragroup communication, training, and cohesion. At all levels of these programs the staff appeared to be highly informed about future plans and felt that they were significantly involved in the decision making process.

Our study and extensive observation of CMHC programs indicate several elements important to policies on planning. First, it seems clear that both time and money must be allocated for this vital stage of program development; and neither should be underestimated, especially if community involvement is deemed important. Since a feeling of ownership by the community promotes support for and use of a CMHC, involving local people in the planning stage provides program staff with invaluable information and advice. Dealing with issues of resource allocation at the initial planning stage of a program alleviates later confusion and misunderstanding.

Program Philosophy

One of the most salient characteristics of the programs we visited was their strong philosophical and ideological focus. In 11 out of the 12 instances, the director described the program as representing a specific philosophy or ideology. Some of these philosophies were concerned with program goals or outcomes, such as keeping patients out of inpatient care by building social support systems; others focused on applying particular techniques or methods such as behavior modification. We found that program philosophy was clearly understood by most of the staff members, and in a few instances clerical staff and even program clients could describe this framework. In one center, a paraprofessional worker described the program director as "the keeper of the principles" and stressed how important these principles were, particularly in guiding the program's future planning. Even in the one program where the project director did not articulate a clear program philosophy, our interviews revealed that the staff shared a large number of ideas and concepts which gave them a sense of identity and helped to focus their work.

This contrasts with the site visitors' experience in other (often less effective) programs where directors tended to describe their programs merely in terms of organizational structure, focusing on numbers of staff, budgets, and expansions. In fact, most mental health center programs are not based on a clearly articulated philosophy. Too often, program directors and staff pay little attention to why the program is doing what it is doing. Staff often have vague and differing philosophies concerning what constitutes mental illness and mental health, and are equally vague in their ideas concerning treatment methods and goals. Such a situation can interfere with the sustained and coordinated efforts required for project success.

A guiding philosophy can make an important contribution to the success of a mental health program in several ways. First, a program philosophy may be viewed as a staff development tool, giving program staff a well-defined basis for making autonomous decisions, resulting in higher levels of individual effort and a better coordination of program activities. Zander (1977), for instance, found group harmony related to group standards. He was not sure which came first, but harmony and standards appear to be interdependent. Second, an articulated philosophy may be viewed as a planning tool, helping to set program goals and evaluate program success. Third, a philosophy may also be a political instrument, helping to prevent ideological splits or divisions within the program and providing a basis for explaining the program to the community.

Bennis (1962) outlined three criteria for organizational health. One of these—a sense of identity—seems to be directly related to program philosophy. If staff hold knowledge and insight about what the ideological premises are and how they can be implemented, and if goals are shared and understood, a program will have a better chance for success. The policy implication is, then, that programs should be urged to articulate a clear philosophy.

Leadership

Eight out of the twelve programs were directed by an individual who was present at its inception. These individuals tended to be strong leaders who saw the program as "their baby" and invested a great deal of time and energy in the process of development. It would be tempting to generalize and suggest that the best program directors were those who had created the ideological and physical foundations of their programs. In many cases this is true, but we also found two instances of programs whose original directors, though deeply committed, lacked the administrative know-how and organizational skills to make the program work. In these cases it was the second generation director who took a faltering program and gave it structure and cohesion. It seems apparent that a successful program director must have a complex array of skills, and that commitment, dedication, and good ideas are not sufficient qualifications for the job if other talents are lacking.

In a recent study of effective technical assistance projects in the field of education, Moore, Schepers, Holmes, and Blair (1977) found that a crucial role of strong leadership is that of entrepreneur. The director must draw together staff, funds, and a tradition of change to develop specific strategies for direct assistance to clients. They also found that while leaders differ in style they were all willing to project a clear direction and to set limits. Our findings in these mental health programs were quite similar.

The directors of the programs we visited had widely varying professional backgrounds. Paraprofessionals with a B.A. degree or less administered five of the programs. The directors of the remaining programs included one M.D., one Ph.D., two R.N.s, and three persons with master's degrees. Paraprofessionals had actually begun three of these programs. In the other cases a professional began the program but later moved a paraprofessional into the day-to-day administrative role. In general, programs with a strong community orientation or those providing services specifically to clients with drug and alcohol problems tended to have less credentialed people as leaders. In several cases the director of the "effective" program we visited was the least credentialed program director in the center. In one instance a great deal of political maneuvering was successfully employed to install as program director a competent person who did not possess the professional (Ph.D. or M.D.) degree usually required to direct a program within a university medical school setting.

In terms of policy, our findings suggest that the leadership of the project is very important to its success in terms of providing a unifying vision and also in terms of the administrative skill necessary to implement that vision. Ability does not seem to be related in any simple way to degree or credentials; requirements for particular degrees for position or advancement do not seem appropriate.

Characteristics of Paraprofessionals

It is difficult to give any precise characterization of such a diverse group of people as paraprofessionals. This section includes a number of general comments and observations about the paraprofessional staff members employed in the programs we visited.

These paraprofessional staff members tended to be warm and easygoing people. Their interpersonal communication skills were well developed; they were equally at ease voicing their feelings and ideas or listening to others'. As a group they had confidence in their skills and competencies, and saw themselves as being genuinely helpful to their clients and communities, feeling a great deal of individual pride in their work and group pride in their programs. In all these programs the paraprofessionals felt that their talents were well used and that their work involved much more than a routine 9:00 to 5:00 job. This is in marked contrast to findings in other programs where paraprofessional staff felt underutilized and thought that they had much more to offer than was asked (Baker, 1972). In such programs morale tended to be lower and there was little sense of pride in the accomplishments of other staff members.

When queried regarding their motives for working as paraprofessionals, virtually all the interviewees mentioned the intrinsic satisfactions of the job. They repeatedly pointed out that they had passed up opportunities to work elsewhere for more pay, but preferred to stay at their present position because of the sense of accomplishment their work gave them. This supports the work of Levinson, Price, Munden, Mandl, and Solley (1962) who found that workers who most closely met their criteria of mental health were those whose work was not merely the means to a paycheck but rather provided "a sense of reward in performing a unique and highly necessary job in a particular community."

Another major source of job satisfaction was the relationships with other staff. Zander (1977) suggests that a strong group shows greater desire for *group* success, and good relations between paraprofessional and other staff certainly encourage this attitude. There was a great deal of group support and rapport in the programs studied. In Likert's (1959) description of highly effective groups he notes:

> The leader and the members believe that each group member can accomplish the "impossible." These expectations stretch each member to the

maximum and accelerate his growth. When necessary, the group tempers
the expectations so that the member is not broken by feelings of failure
or rejection.

It seems likely that in these high stress jobs group support is important
to guard against the syndrome of frustration and exhaustion known as burning
out. In fact, we observed a number of situations in which a paraprofessional
used peer support to cope with a particularly difficult problem. In one case a
staff member came into the central office, very upset because of an attempted
suicide by her client. The other staff listened attentively and sympathetically,
shared similar experiences, joked with her, and ended up taking her to lunch.
Such support in times of crisis very probably enables staff to take on more
responsibility than would otherwise be possible.

The question of salaries, particularly paraprofessionals' versus professionals' salaries, was a persistent point of friction. Nearly all paraprofessionals
considered their wages to be too low and incommensurate with their responsibilities. While they generally did not object to professionals' salaries being
higher, they did feel that the differential was too great.

Paraprofessionals in mental health come from a wide variety of backgrounds, and this makes it difficult to generalize in any discussion of the
paraprofessionals' previous experiences. We did note, however, that the paraprofessionals in the programs studied tended to be drawn from three different
groups.

One group was composed of young people with college experience either
at a four-year institution or a junior college. Such college experience, whether
or not a degree is obtained, seems to leave the students with a desire for further
schooling and also a need for a worthwhile occupation. When such people
become paraprofessionals they see their work as a chance for a meaningful
experience and an opportunity to explore the mental health field as a career.
Many of these people plan to eventually obtain further professional training.
They seem to reflect a trend toward the employment of better educated paraprofessionals with a more middle-class background, and away from the employment of ex-clients or indigenous paraprofessionals. One reason for this
trend might be the employment situation in the 1970s, which impels many
people with B.A.s and even M.A.s to apply for paraprofessional positions. It
is possible that professional staff members in a position to influence hiring
decisions may feel more comfortable with paraprofessionals who come from
a similar background. It is also true that the 1960s New Careers ideology,
which stressed employment of individuals from poverty backgrounds, has
faded, in part because of diminished federal support.

In spite of this trend there is still a large group of paraprofessionals drawn
from indigenous or poverty groups and serving those populations. These paraprofessionals have the advantage of special knowledge of the community because of their residence within it or ethnic identification with it. In some

programs a paraprofessional from a minority or poverty background was selected with the general intention of bringing a fresh perspective to the middle-class-oriented professional staff; in other cases indigenous staff helped the program in specific ways by bridging language and cultural barriers within the community. In none of the programs we visited was the hiring of indigenous staff merely tokenism or political; these people were not present for window dressing but were genuinely useful because of their special knowledge.

There was a third, smaller group of paraprofessionals consisting of people who had dealt successfully with specific psychological problems within themselves, such as alcoholism, drug dependency, and mental illness. It has been common practice in programs serving alcoholics and drug users to hire paraprofessionals who have themselves overcome such problems. In a few other programs ex-mental patients have been hired. In all these cases the paraprofessionals serve as role models, demonstrating to clients that their difficulties can indeed be overcome and giving first-hand information regarding how this might be accomplished.

More and more colleges are establishing A.A. and B.A. programs in mental health and human service. Our own research indicates that over 300 such programs now exist (Alley & Blanton, 1978). The existence of these formal training programs provides an impetus for mental health and human service agencies to raise educational standards for their paraprofessional employees. The increases in educational standards in turn generate a demand for more training programs.

Certainly college training programs can increase the skills that staff bring to agencies and can decrease the necessity for large in-service training programs. On the other hand, too much reliance on college training has its hazards and may even subvert important purposes for paraprofessional employment. Excessive reliance on middle-class paraprofessionals with traditional academic backgrounds can produce an inadequate representation of minority staff, those from poverty backgrounds, and those who have overcome their own personal mental health problems. In terms of policy, agencies should not require A.A. or B.A. degrees as a screening for potential employees.

Agency staff and the paraprofessionals themselves complain that some of the college programs do not prepare paraprofessionals for the tasks and problems that they find on the job. Academic training is not the only route to acquisition of the skills which are required of paraprofessionals. Life experience, in-service training, and on-the-job supervision should be seen as legitimate alternatives to classroom instruction. In the minds of many paraprofessionals and their supervisors these alternatives may even prove, in some cases, to be superior.

In order to provide adequate training for those paraprofessionals who do not enter with sufficient training (whether college educated or not), the agencies must allocate specific resources to the development and implementation of a good training/supervision system. Such a system would include in-house training as well as incentives (funds, time) for staff to continue their job-related education.

A third policy suggestion would be to urge degree programs to allow credit for in-service training, on-the-job supervision, and life experience. Model programs such as this currently exist at the University of Oregon and the College for Human Service in New York. These processes would allow paraprofessionals alternate routes to learning, job mobility, and promotion.

In order to achieve an appropriate balance of staff, policymakers should examine selection requirements to make sure that educational standards are not set at arbitrarily high levels, to allow alternate routes of upward mobility through in-service or on-the-job training, to allow substitution of appropriate documented experience for college training, and to allocate funds for staff development and training of special population groups.

Program Structure

The programs we visited tended to have rather uncomplicated organizational structures, having only two or three rank levels between the program director and the lowest ranking paraprofessional. This unelaborate hierarchy was probably related to organizational size, which tended to be less than 30 staff. The informal structure tended to be even flatter than the formal structure. For example, the project director, the staff psychiatrists, and other professionals were usually accessible to the other, lower-ranking staff. Levinson et al. (1962) have suggested that good relations between staff and supervisory personnel require that supervisors not just be "good guys," but that they know the work, plan it well, keep staff informed, and be reliable. Although Levinson was referring to supervisors in a gas and electric company, these standards seem to hold for the mental health organizations studied here.

In more than half the sites visited, the division of work did not strictly follow traditional, professional roles. In other words, merely knowing that a staff person was a social worker, psychologist, psychiatrist, nurse, or paraprofessional would not automatically reveal what these people actually did. While psychologists tended to do most of the testing and psychiatrists were the only staff members to prescribe medications, there was a great deal of overlap in terms of who did counseling, outreach, running of groups, administration, consultation, and training. Paraprofessionals were involved in all these activities. And in all but one program, paraprofessionals had a voice in determining the design of their jobs and the nature of their duties.

Clients in the programs we visited frequently were assigned to individual staff members, professional or paraprofessional, who were in charge throughout the clients' involvement in the programs; this facilitated continuity of care and required that staff members be familiar with a wide variety of treatment options. As opposed to clinical settings where individual therapists derive their sense of success from the progress of their individual clients, these program staff seemed to see their work as highly interrelated. Zander (1977) discussed groups that create "products" attributed to the unit as a whole, not to particular members. The staff with whom we spoke had some sense of working both for themselves and for the larger group. If Zander's assumptions are correct this might contribute to the strengths of the group and promote greater desire for group success.

The programs we visited were subunits of a larger center in all but one instance. In seven of the programs a substantial amount of program activity took place away from the parent center, either at satellite clinics or in the community as outreach work. In some cases this situation tended to cause an "us-them" attitude to develop between such programs and the rest of the center. In two cases this eventually provoked a crisis so severe that the center director felt it necessary to physically move the program to "bring it closer" to the rest of the center. At first these findings surprised us, since we had assumed that these exemplary programs would be well integrated within the parent organization. We found that the programs did indeed have good referral mechanisms connecting them with the rest of the center but clearly had a sense of their own separate identities.

Moore (1977) and his colleagues have pointed out the strains of geographic dispersion. Policy must anticipate the difficulties inherent in relations between parent centers and individual programs and focus on the process of the interdependence between the two.

Program Functioning

Although recruitment tended to be informal and unsystematic, the selection of staff was considered to be extremely important in every program we visited. Interestingly, only two of the programs were involved with a rigid civil service type of recruitment, and both programs had developed loopholes to provide more flexibility in hiring. In all but one case the paraprofessional staff were involved in the selection of professional staff.

Characteristics generally deemed important in the selection of paraprofessional employees included flexibility, warmth, ability to handle stress, and previous experience in working with people. Selection of professional staff focused on the prospective staff members' ability to fit into the group as well as their competence. This bias is similar to the findings of Lewis (1975) who studied college teacher selection and found that ability to get along with others was more important in selection than talent or productivity. In one program a new professional was to be hired, and the staff chose a younger, less experienced applicant instead of a more experienced person because the applicant selected "seemed to be a part of the group." This "fraternity" system of selection may be particularly useful in programs that are small and rely on group cohesion to prevent burn out.

In some of the programs there was little or no turnover in staff. Scott (1965) found that groups that favored recruitment of individuals "like us" held members longer and exhibited greater organizational stability. Our observations support this view. In other programs, paraprofessional staff tended to stay about two years and then leave. In these latter cases there was little or no possibility for upward mobility for staff, and workers had to move to other agencies in order to receive a higher salary or have more responsibility. In the programs with little turnover, the staff seemed to have a better chance for increased pay and responsibility or felt deeply committed to the program and were not interested in a different sort of job even if it paid more.

We were surprised to find that, with a few notable exceptions, the programs we visited seldom implemented formal training programs. Most training involved a general orientation and then an informal apprenticeship with another staff member. This buddy system of training was supplemented with some in-service training programs which tended to consist of a loosely coordinated group of lectures and seminars on interesting or relevant topics. Most staff members seemed to believe that learning was a by-product of doing and that on-the-job experience with supervision was the best type of instruction.

We were also surprised to find that, with a few exceptions, these effective programs generally had weak and inefficient evaluation systems. Since most mental health programs tend to be weak in this area, we believe that these effective programs are merely reflecting this general tendency. Staff members tended to see evaluation as a low priority and sometimes complained that it interfered with their direct services to clients. In general, demographic and process records were kept, but little effort was given to formal, ongoing assessment of client progress, program impact, or staff performance. One center gathered an enormous amount of data and had a highly sophisticated computer system, but the system was so cumbersome that it was seldom used for decision making.

There were a few notable exceptions to the general lack of properly functioning evaluation systems. The behavior modification program's evaluation was a model of efficiency, not only in data gathering but in its use of data to provide feedback to clients and evaluation of client progress and staff effectiveness. Another program with an effective evaluation system suggested that it was difficult to introduce an evaluation system after the program was in operation and advised programs to design their evaluation system prior to hiring staff members so evaluation and recordkeeping would be seen by them, from the outset, as part of their job responsibility. Generally, program staff members found evaluation more acceptable if it actually helped them in their service delivery functions by giving them useful feedback concerning their job performance and the progress of clients.

These findings have some policy implications. Adherence to rigid civil service type requirements in staff selection may reduce the ability of programs to select individuals who work well as part of a team. If team cohesion does indeed contribute to better morale and productivity, then it may be necessary to allow greater flexibility in hiring. Scriven (1978) talks about hiring in terms of merit (traditional civil service procedures) and in terms of value (benefit to the institution). More careful attention to both must be considered when selecting mental health staff. In order to foster organizational stability and low staff turnover, policies should be explored which would provide paraprofessional staff with the possibility of career mobility, increased responsibility, and regulated pay increases. Careful analysis of the formal and informal training needs within a center must be made. In general, evaluations need to be strengthened, particularly models which provide service staff with useful ongoing feedback about the progress of their clients and their own performance.

Program Climate

When compared with other human service programs we have visited in which intragroup antagonism was frequent, the relationships in this sample of effective programs were strikingly cordial. In every case the project director was well liked and respected. This positive regard may have been instrumental in generating the high degree of commitment we observed in the staff regarding project philosophy and goals. At all the sites we visited the director had a strong commitment to the use of paraprofessionals and made this commitment known not only to the staff but to the parent center and the community. The staff also felt that the director respected their work. The contrast is notable between these findings, which are representative of highly successful programs, and information from a more heterogeneous sample of programs studied by Baker (1972), who found that paraprofessionals often feel that they are not appreciated or understood by the professional staff.

While positive feelings predominated, site visitors were also struck by the open and frank manner in which the staff would criticize each other, the project, and the director. In all sites staff characterized the project as open to criticism. Levinson et al. (1962) noted that the constructive handling of problems by supervisory personnel decreased stress within organizations. They indicated that effective leaders openly recognize organizational problems, demonstrate some understanding of employee difficulties, and mobilize staff efforts in seeking solutions to problems. While confrontations and disagreements did occur in the programs studied (perhaps with greater frequency than in other programs we have visited), disputes tended to concern genuine service issues rather than petty or narrowly personal matters, and these issues were handled promptly and forthrightly, generally with some satisfactory resolution.

In many mental health centers we have visited, the paraprofessional staff and the professional staff interacted very little, either at work or socially. This contrasts sharply with these effective programs where there was a great deal of informal social contact between the professionals and the paraprofessionals. These programs seem to have achieved what Levinson et al. (1962) have termed a "balanced distance." This concept describes the tension between inappropriate intimacy among members of an organization and too much distance. Staff members in all programs, for instance, felt that they received needed emotional support from other staff, both professional and paraprofessional. Straight talk seemed to be the rule, and this was paired with genuine affection and respect shared among staff.

While policy cannot legislate a healthy program climate, concrete kinds of evaluation systems and review procedures can be designed and implemented that will allow problems to surface and be dealt with in a constructive manner.

Summary

To review the common characteristics shared by these effective programs: The programs studied tended to do substantial planning prior to the onset of the program and to continue planning on an ongoing basis. Community people as well as professionals were often involved in planning procedures. Staff selection did not focus on formal credentials but on competence and ability to fit into the group. Compared with other programs within the same center, the staff of these programs often had fewer credentials. The programs generally had a unifying philosophical stance, and staff felt a strong sense of group identity and pride in what the program was accomplishing for clients. Top level staff tended to be accessible to all levels of staff, and in general the communication between staff members was quite considerable and open.

A brief survey of some theories of organizational effectiveness can be set against our findings of these effective programs employing paraprofessionals. Bennis (1962) modified Jahoda's (1958) formulations about individual mental health and outlined three criteria for organizational health: (1) adaptability, (2) a sense of identity, and (3) the capacity to test reality. Levinson's concept of "flexibility under stress" seems more appropriate to community mental health center programs than the mere "adaptability" suggested by Bennis. Argyris (1964) added a fourth criterion: the integration among subparts of the total organization such that parts are not working at crosspurposes. Since paraprofessionals are the lowest paid and most numerous of mental health providers, their successful integration within mental health programs may be a bellwether for the overall health of the organization.

Levinson's (1962) concept of reciprocity and interdependence between the worker and the organization also seems to be an important factor in making the work environment more conducive to the mental health of the worker. It is difficult to imagine that staff who are dissatisfied and defensive, who feel unappreciated, and who hold little pride or sense of identity with their work could provide high quality treatment to mental health clients. Finally, Blake and Mouton (1964) assert that organizational effectiveness is achieved when management succeeds in being both production and person centered. In mental health organizations the product itself (mental health services) can be considered to be person centered. Thus the importance of personal relations within this type of organization might have particular significance. More information is certainly needed on interstaff relations and their effect on client services.

The trends found in these effective programs suggest areas for further systematic study. They also may provide clues which program planners and administrators can use to assist them in improving their organizational functioning.

REFERENCES

Alley, S. R., & Blanton, J. *Report to NIMH Contract #NEC 1 T31 MH 15414–01,* September 1978.

Argyris, C. *Integrating the individual and the organization.* New York: John Wiley, 1964.

Baker, E. J. The mental health associate: A new approach in mental health. *Community Mental Health Journal,* 1972, *8,* 281–291.

Bennis, W. G. Toward a "truly" scientific management: The concept of organizational health. *General Systems Yearbook,* 1962, *7,* 271–296.

Blake, R. R., & Mouton, J. *The managerial grid.* Houston, Tex.: Gulf Publishing, 1964.

Blanton, J., & Alley, S. Models of program success in New Careers programs. *Journal of Community Psychology,* 1977, *5,* 359–371.

Jahoda, M. *Current concepts of positive mental health.* New York: Basic Books, 1958.

Levinson, H., Price, C. R., Munden, K. J., Mandl, H. J., & Solley, C. M. *Men, management, and mental health.* Cambridge, Mass.: Harvard University Press, 1962.

Lewis, L. S. *Scaling the ivory tower.* Baltimore: Johns Hopkins University Press, 1975.

Likert, R. *New patterns of management.* New York: McGraw Hill, 1961.

Moore, D. R., Schepers, E. M., Holmes, M. L., & Blair, K. A. *Summary: Assistance strategies of six groups that facilitate educational change at the school/community level* (Final Report, National Institute of Education Project No. 4–0768). Chicago: Center for New Schools, 1977.

Scott, W. *Values and organizations.* Chicago: Rand McNally, 1965.

Scriven, M. *Evaluation News,* 1978, *6,* (August).

Zander, A. *Groups at work.* San Francisco: Jossey-Bass, 1977.

SUPERVISION

The supervision of staff members by qualified personnel is a valuable quality control and training strategy in any community mental health service area. Supervision is especially important in all services where staff members and clients carry out an extended series of relatively autonomous one-to-one interactions that may have a significant impact on the client's well-being.

For these reasons, we decided to describe in more detail one particular approach to the supervision of paraprofessionals; the approach is carried out, in this case, in an outpatient program. This method involves using supervision as a training strategy and is particularly appropriate for paraprofessionals without preservice training or prior supervised clinical experience. The supervising professionals are skilled *both* as therapists and as teacher-supervisors.

The outpatient program chosen for this purpose is a division of the Hahnemann Community Mental Health Center in Philadelphia.* The Hahnemann Center is affiliated with the Hahnemann Medical College. A sizable majority of outpatient therapists (whether professional or paraprofessional) receive individual supervision from senior medical school faculty and consultants and/or from the medical directors of the satellite clinics in which they work. In addition, all outpatient therapists receive group supervision.

*Contact: Hahnemann Community Mental Health Center
314 North Broad
Philadelphia, Pennsylvania 19102
215/568-0860
Attention: Edward Volkman, Director of Outpatient Services

The paraprofessionals at Hahnemann are primarily natives of Philadelphia and the surrounding area, and the majority of them are members of ethnic minority groups. They help to expand the range of services that Hahnemann is able to provide and the number of people reached through the services. Furthermore, the paraprofessionals broaden the cultural relevance of the services and make services psychologically more accessible to the consumers. Since 1971, a sizable percentage of new paraprofessional therapists hired by the center have been graduates of the medical college's two-year training program for mental health technologists; enrolling at the A.A. level, the students are graduated with B.S. degrees. Some of the program's paraprofessionals, however, have not received this university-based training. (In 1976, the medical college initiated a two-year training program that emphasizes preventive strategies; the graduates of this new program receive A.A. degress.)

This appendix is based on interviews with both the senior medical school supervisors and with the paraprofessional outpatient therapists. These interviews dealt with general features of supervision as well as with the needs and characteristics of the paraprofessional staff members who had been hired without extensive prior training. The material presented here represents a blending of the viewpoints expressed by the supervising professional staff members and by the paraprofessional personnel.

BRIEF DESCRIPTION OF THE CENTER AND PROGRAM

The Hahnemann Center is located in the middle of Philadelphia and serves the 130,000 residents of one of the most impoverished sections of Pennsylvania. About 55% of the residents are black; another 15 to 18% are Puerto Rican. Outpatient services are delivered in seven facilities scattered throughout the catchment area. Under Pennsylvania laws, mental health centers can be reimbursed for outpatient services delivered by paraprofessionals; 90% of the catchment area residents are eligible for income-related coverage. Anthony A. Arce, M.D., directs the center, while Edward Volkman, M.D., leads the outpatient program.

Professional and most paraprofessional outpatient therapists perform the same service functions. To perform a given function, however, paraprofessionals must demonstrate a command of the relevant competencies; all paraprofessionals are given supervised opportunities to demonstrate their expertise. The functions that paraprofessionals can perform include: intake evaluations, individual therapy, therapy by pairs of clinicians (cotherapy), family and group therapy, emergency room shifts, helping clients with daily living needs, and paying home visits. Both professional and paraprofessional staff members do the same things, except that the paraprofessionals tend to devote a somewhat higher percentage of their time to the latter two functions. Supervision for the paraprofessionals is concentrated on the areas where the paraprofessionals have less knowledge.

The satellite clinics operate under a dual leadership system. A psychiatrist in each clinic is a medical director, responsible for clinical concerns; a nonpsychiatrist in each clinic is an administrator, responsible for nonclinical administrative matters. The administrator of one of the satellite clinics is a paraprofessional; this paraprofessional is also a therapist. In the therapeutic role, the paraprofessional is supervised without role-related problems by a professional staff member who is administratively "under the paraprofessional's command."

The clients seen at the clinics are often overwhelmed by the circumstances of their lives, and so they tend to require assistance in daily living needs. Frequently, they do not keep appointments. For these reasons, long-term verbal therapy is not always appropriate or practical as a first service to clients. When providing services to clients, staff members accordingly often focus initially on the client's concrete concerns (e.g., finding a job, resolving an interpersonal conflict), and only later does the therapist shift to more abstract, underlying issues. The typical client sees a staff member on perhaps 15 occasions, spread over a 5 to 6 month period.

The paraprofessional staff members perform concrete functions. By helping a client to receive welfare or to find a suitable lawyer, for example, a clinician can establish a relationship of trust with a client. In addition, by alleviating the client's basic needs, the therapist can prepare a client to profit the most from future formalized therapy services from the same or other clinicians. Flexible work hours make it possible for staff clinicians to provide concrete services to clients, for these services are often carried out outside of the 8:00 a.m. to 5:00 p.m., Monday through Friday work week. The program is not reimbursed by third party payments for "nontherapy" work, but the administrative staff members prefer to provide a wide array of services rather than to focus only on services for which third party reimbursement is available.

SUPERVISION

General Features of Supervision

The senior supervisors all hold faculty appointments at the Hahnemann Medical College. These senior supervisors include the director of the Hahnemann Center, the director of the outpatient program, the medical directors of each satellite clinic, both the director of residency training and the chairman of the department of psychiatry from the medical college, and a consulting psychoanalyst. The professional staff members from the outpatient program also supervise the paraprofessionals. The vast majority of paraprofessionals receive approximately 1 to 2 hours of one-to-one case-oriented supervision weekly from these various professionals. Furthermore, paraprofessionals receive 2 to 4 hours of group supervision weekly from senior supervisors and other professionals.

Supervision as a Training Strategy

Two Functions of Supervision.   Supervision is used at the Hahnemann Center both to evaluate and to train new paraprofessionals. Supervisors who are employed as part of the center staff tend to emphasize the evaluative function. As the paraprofessionals become more competent, these supervisors place increasing emphasis on the supervisory function as a training strategy. The supervisors who are hired as consultants from outside the center primarily use supervision as a training strategy. Supervisors are deliberately rotated, so that the paraprofessionals can receive training from a changing array of professionals.

Paraprofessionals can use the supervisory time to discuss various specific crises met during the week. Supervisors encourage the paraprofessionals to ask questions, and emphasize the appropriateness of asking a more experienced person to take over a difficult case. To aid in teaching, however, the supervisors generally spend the entire session on a single case. This approach makes it possible to cover the issues in greater depth. Because the paraprofessionals have many clients, the supervisors discuss different individual cases during different weeks.

Overcoming Communication Barriers. Both senior supervisors and paraprofessionals mentioned that the paraprofessionals tend to be ill-at-ease in group supervisory sessions. For some paraprofessionals this lack of ease may also be present in one-to-one supervisory sessions, especially if the supervisor makes considerable use of technical terminology. A contributing cause is the fact that inexperienced therapists (whether professional or paraprofessional) encounter difficulty in describing in fine detail the events that have occurred while therapy and other services are being provided to clients. Over a period of time this skill improves, as the supervisees learn to use the supervisory sessions effectively and as a result of the training conditions established by supervisors.

One senior supervisor described supervision as "metatherapy," as therapy for therapists. The goal of the supervisor is to develop a feeling of trust with the paraprofessionals and to assist the paraprofessionals in learning to rely on their own resources. For supervisors, a major route for achieving these goals is to discuss specific issues in a supportive fashion.

One relevant approach is to videotape a paraprofessional's therapy sessions for the purpose of subsequent viewing and discussion. This procedure enables the supervisor and paraprofessional to discuss the concrete behavior both of the client and the therapist. These discussions can be used to help the paraprofessional to learn the vocabulary for describing therapeutic interchanges; as a result, the paraprofessional can be more relaxed in supervisory sessions. The discussions also allow supervisors to see the paraprofessional's behavior and to help the paraprofessional to set realistic expectations as a clinician. Another relevant approach is to team a supervisor and a paraprofessional as cotherapits. Initially, the supervisor will probably make most of the therapeutic interventions. By observing the supervisor and from the discussions that occur upon the completion of each therapy session, the paraprofessional learns helpful therapeutic strategies. As a result, the paraprofessional is gradually able to assume more responsibility for the therapeutic interactions.

The paraprofessional staff members reported that the supervisory relationship is enhanced if the supervisors are willing to learn from them. One paraprofessional described a particularly able supervisor who learned about the community from the paraprofessional during the supervisory sessions. Supervisors can also be more effective with paraprofessionals if they show their concern for a client by helping the paraprofessional to deal with a case in concrete ways. A paraprofessional described a situation in which the supervisor accompanied the paraprofessional on a home visit and thus was able to understand the case better and give more helpful support. In order to gain a clearer understanding of a case, at the Hahnemann Center a supervisor occasionally spends an hour with a client with whom a paraprofessional is experiencing difficulty.

Specific Difficulties that Supervision Can Prevent

Erroneous Assessments. It was reported that clients are often most comfortable receiving therapy from the clinician whom they meet during the intake session. However, paraprofessionals (especially if they have not attended an extensive preservice training program) do not always perform accurate intake assessments. Some paraprofessionals have particular difficulty in diagnosing situations where medication is appropriate, in identifying the possible underlying motivations for behavior, and in determining when clients may be predisposed to violent or suicidal behavior. Errors in the original assessment of a client can be detected and corrected through the case-centered discussions that occur in the context of one-to-one supervision of the paraprofessional and in case conferences. The paraprofessional can learn how to assess a client's treatment needs by performing the intake evaluation collaboratively with the supervising professionals.

Because the novice therapist may have the tendency to focus on surface behavior, paraprofessionals may inappropriately interpret a client's verbal behavior as exclusively manipulative. For example, a paraprofessional may react personally to a client's lying, rather than dealing with why the client is lying. A similar focus on surface behavior can cause paraprofessionals to underestimate the seriousness of the symptoms of psychosis. For example, a paraprofessional may interpret a client's talk of suicide as a problem which can be alleviated by convincing the client to stop mentioning the subject. In actuality, however, the client may suffer from a deep-seated lack of control that causes a genuine predisposition to commit suicide. One difficulty in teaching paraprofessionals to focus on the underlying motives of the client's behavior is that the paraprofessionals may overestimate their understanding of the clients' problems because of their similar backgrounds.

Inappropriate Treatment Strategies.   Paraprofessionals lacking in extensive preservice training may believe that a good heart and conscientious effort are sufficient to cure a client. The paraprofessionals may not realize that they may undermine the client's autonomy by offering excessive assistance, or that their natural warmth and supportiveness are not always in the client's best interests. Through a process of supervision by more experienced personnel, the paraprofessional can learn to say "no" to unreasonable or self-defeating requests from clients and to come up with treatment plans that allow a client to become more autonomous.

Paraprofessional staff members who are unconvinced of the importance of a theoretical framework may emphasize pragmatic results rather than the development of a treatment plan that deals with a client's underlying problems. The example given previously about suicidal statements is a case in point. However, some clients are more interested in concrete solutions to problems than in an understanding of the underlying dynamics of their problems. The tendency of some paraprofessionals to focus on surface behavior, thus, can be in accord with the desires of some clients. For these clients an ideal treatment strategy for paraprofessionals to employ might entail assistance with concrete concerns; the paraprofessionals' interventions, however, should be based on an understanding of the underlying motives.

In Conclusion

At the Hahnemann Community Mental Health Center supervision is used systematically as a training strategy, as well as to evaluate the performance of salaried staff members. The supervisors use a variety of approaches to establish relationships with supervisees that are based on mutual trust and learning. As a result, the quality of services to clients is enhanced, especially in regard to the reduction in frequency of erroneous assessments and inappropriate treatment strategies.

IMPLEMENTATION OF PROGRAM IDEAS

Organizational change and the diffusion of ideas are complex processes, not easily reduced to simple recipes. Writing about alternative programs does not of itself lead others to organize and implement such programs. We hope that reading the 12 case studies may be a first step toward effecting positive change in a mental health organization. If you are interested in adapting some aspect of one of the models described in this volume to a particular program, the following suggestions may be helpful.

For each program, the full mailing address and telephone number are given on the first page of the chapter, making it possible to contact the program for futher discussion of interesting ideas.

The Paraprofessional Manpower Branch, National Institute of Mental Health, Parklawn Building, 5600 Fishers Lane, Rockville, Maryland 20852, may be contacted for information about service programs making effective use of paraprofessionals and on special training programs oriented towards paraprofessionals. The staff members of this office are also informed about current resources in the paraprofessional field.

The Social Action Research Center, 2728 Durant Avenue, Berkeley, California 94704, may be contacted to provide information of a similar nature as well as assistance in problems of planning and making changes within an organization. The Social Action Research Center has also prepared additional literature, including a fully annotated bibliography (Social Action Rescarch Center, 1977) containing more than 1,300 entries, which are cross-indexed by category and by author, concerning the use of paraprofessionals in community mental health. The companion book to this volume, *Paraprofessionals in Mental Health: Theory and Practice* (Alley, Blanton, & Feldman, Note 1) contains chapters discussing various issues that relate to paraprofessional use. The chapter entitled "A Guide to the Indigenous Change Agent," by Louis Tornatsky, is especially appropriate to assist in organizational change.

Howard Davis, Chief, Mental Health Services Development Branch, NIMH, has developed an organizational change model, represented by the acronym A VICTORY, which raises important questions organizational staff must answer before planning to introduce change (Larsen & Norris, 1977).

> *Abilities:* Do we have the abilities, the resources, and capabilities?
>
> *Values:* Does the new program match the values, the style, and philosophy of our institution?
>
> *Information:* What and where is the information we need to consider and then implement the new program?
>
> *Circumstances:* What circumstances must we consider in the environment occupied by our agency?
>
> *Timing:* How's the timing? Is now the right time to do it?
>
> *Obligation:* Is there an obligation to change? Why change at all?
>
> *Resistances:* What resistances might we expect?
>
> *Yields:* What yields can we expect from the change?

In the course of our research over the past year, we had occasion to discuss with the staff members and administration of five of our effective programs detailed ideas concerning strategies for implementing a program such as theirs in another setting. What follows in this appendix are the results of these discussions in the areas of Children's Services, Follow-up Services, Outpatient Services, and Screening Services. Much of what is written might be generalized to additional service areas.

Ideas for Implementing a Children's Program

A children's program in the tradition of the Huntsville-Madison County Community Mental Health Center would apply an objective, accountable approach to service delivery, and thus would use ongoing evaluation procedures and emphasize competency. The administrative procedures required for offering rewards to employees for competent performance can probably be better carried out in a small- or medium-sized organization. It is important that the community board and center director be dedicated to accountability and that the professionals in power be receptive to implementing a program that rewards and recognizes paraprofessionals and professionals alike for enhanced professional competencies.

It is probably more difficult to change an existing program over to the behavior modification tradition than to begin a new program. The Huntsville Center had been traditional in its service delivery and accountability practices prior to 1971, when the changeover to the behavior modification model took place. During the first three years of the "new regime" a sizable percentage of employees (about 35%) resigned each year. The new evaluation procedures were the target of many employee complaints, and probably contributed to the high turnover rate.

In changing an existing center to the behavior modification model, it is important to use an approach of "successive approximations" to the final goal. An example might be the introduction of the new evaluation procedures. First, a process should be developed to hold the director(s) accountable for their own performance. Only after the director(s) have taken this initiative should staff members be expected to participate. Second, the center should be shut down, if possible, for intensive staff orientation and training. It would be desirable for the center to secure funding for developing the needed in-service training program.

The general public may be hostile toward behavior modification approaches because of some widely publicized abuses by behavior modification practitioners, or those claiming to be behavior therapists. Such hostility can be reduced if the center emphasizes accountability and pragmatism (that the approach works) rather than techniques. In Huntsville, the behavioral approach is now accepted widely in the community, even by conservative members of the clergy. The acceptance comes in large measure from successful experiences with behavior modification by clients, relatives of clients, consultees, and professionals, and from the resulting informal discussions of these experiences with other residents of the catchment area. Moreover, the use of technical jargon when describing behavioral principles has been studiously avoided.

Evaluation functions require about 10% of staff time in a center dedicated to accountability and objectivity. Such centers should provide necessary resources, including a separate research and evaluation service that centralizes evaluation activities and reduces duplication of efforts. Furthermore, the children's program (and other center programs) should employ an administrator and a staff to carry out the program's evaluation activities.

A day treatment division within a children's program should be careful not to duplicate services already being received from public agencies (e.g., schools) by catchment area children. Otherwise, the program may experience difficulty in securing reimbursements for these school-related services. If a consultation and education division within a children's program employs behavior modification practices, it should demonstrate these practices to community agencies making requests for case consultation. Agencies are more likely to become enthusiastic about behavior modification after seeing that agency clients have been helped by the approach.

Paraprofessionals in a Children's Program.   Paraprofessionals in the Huntsville program provide competent service at a lower cost than would be possible solely with professional staff members. Their competent performance depends upon a carefully constructed and consistently implemented system of training, supervision, and evaluation procedures. The employee orientation training itself requires some eight weeks for completion. The training program developed by the Huntsville Center is appropriate to paraprofessionals who possess rather high verbal skills. While taking Huntsville's training program for new staff, A.A.-level paraprofessionals might require more time for training than would baccalaureate-level paraprofessionals.

The use of paraprofessionals in working or communicating with community professionals depends on both the role the paraprofessional plays and community attitudes and expectations regarding that role. In such tasks as keeping a judge informed about the progress of a child referred to the day treatment center, a paraprofessional worker would probably not encounter problems. However, paraprofessionals engaging in roles traditionally reserved for professionals (e.g., school consultation) will be more successful if special efforts are made to assure community professionals of the competence of the paraprofessionals. And in certain roles, such as providing court testimony, profes-

sionals are used in Huntsville in preference to paraprofessionals because of local attitudes. For similar reasons, professionals are more effective in such tasks as assuring
distraught parents that their child is not "crazy" and in interpreting tests on which this
assurance may be based.

Ideas for Implementing a Consultation and Education (C & E) Program

The suggestions and recommendations made in this section are most relevant to C &
E programs that form a separate program within a community mental health center,
and those having a strong focus on equal-status working relationships between professional and paraprofessional staff members.

The C & E Program and the Community.   Staff members at the Dr. Solomon
Carter Fuller Mental Health Center believed that the C & E program should be the
first service division established in a new center. The C & E program can then be used
as a vehicle for determining community needs, and for communicating these needs to
the direct service programs. The ideas described in this section, however, can also be
applied to a C & E program within an established community mental health center.

Both paraprofessionals and professionals require training in the mental health
consultation and education skills that should be applied in community settings. Neither
long-term membership in a community nor academic training can guarantee the competent application or the full comprehension of these complex procedures. In addition,
a C & E in-service training program ideally would include some coverage of the direct
services relevant to the consultation and education services provided to clients. For
example, a consultant to a community agency that primarily offers counseling services
should have some grounding in therapeutic principles and techniques.

Program-centered consultation is usually initiated by the Fuller C & E services
through center or program publicity efforts. The organizations approve of this method
of initiating contact. These findings suggest that a C & E program should publicize itself
in the community, and follow up publicity-education efforts with active initiation of
service contacts. It should be noted that agencies sometimes approach the C & E
program with requests for consultative services; a C & E program should be equipped
to respond with reasonable speed to these requests.

The C & E Program and Its Center.   A C & E program should implement
procedures for maintaining both autonomy from and collaboration with other center
programs. Unfortunately, these goals are not always compatible at the outset. The
maintenance of autonomy may interfere temporarily with the achievement of collaboration.

The director of the C & E program will ideally possess sufficient status to give the
director (and thus the program) considerable influence within the center and community. Academic appointments at institutions of higher education can be especially useful
in this respect, regardless of whether the center itself is affiliated with a university. In
the Fuller Center, both C & E directors possessed additional qualities necessary for
effective performance of their responsibilities including familiarity with the community,
organizing skills, political consciousness, and personal resilience.

For the sake of autonomy, it may be preferable for a C & E program to have a
budget administered separately from the parent center's budget. However, if the C &

E funds are disbursed by the center, then the C & E program and the center should formulate written guidelines concerning the C & E activities which the center will commit itself to support. In the absence of such a firm commitment, a center may yield to pressure to increase direct services, and as a consequence may neglect C & E efforts.

C & E program staff members need to educate other center staff members concerning C & E activities. Collaborative efforts between the C & E unit and other units in work-related projects are also useful in improving communication and promoting mutual respect and cooperation. For example, while a C & E program may be primarily responsible for program-centered consultation given to community organizations, it may also collaborate with the center's direct service programs in providing case-centered consultation services to agencies.

The Introduction of Change.   In any program that actually practices participatory decision-making, basic changes tend to occur slowly. The involvement of all staff members takes time, but if a basic change is forced on a program's staff without extensive prior discussion, the program's egalitarian atmosphere, community orientation, and morale may suffer.

In setting up a new C & E program, it is probably advisable to develop and introduce relevant organizational features before beginning actual operations. For example, supervisory procedures may be very difficult to introduce in an ongoing C & E program. If supervision is required in a new program, this procedure should be introduced at the outset. Similarly, planning, staffing, and evaluation-monitoring procedures are more easily implemented if they are built into the program at the time of its inception.

Paraprofessionals in a C & E Program.   In implementing a C & E model such as that in the Fuller program, representatives of the community should play a major role in the selection of staff members, including the director. Community representation in the hiring process should be supplemented by community representation on the actual C & E staff. Paraprofessionals are essential for a C & E program wishing to pursue the goals of the Fuller program. Paraprofessionals who are indigenous to the community, and therefore represent the people who live in the community, help to link the community with the center. Furthermore, paraprofessionals can identify sources of community strength, aid in pinpointing and alleviating community needs, and work well in community settings. In addition, they can transmit these skills to program professionals.

If funds for paying paraprofessionals are not available, then a "critical mass" of community volunteers can be substituted. Whether working as volunteer or paid staff, paraprofessionals should receive the same privileges, power, and respect that are accorded to staff professionals, as well as opportunities for promotions and upgrading of their jobs.

Ideas for Implementing a Follow-up Program

Qualifications for the Program Director.   In order to implement a follow-up model similar to that of the ACS program of the Cambridge-Somerville Mental Health and Retardation Center, the program director should be a skilled clinician in addition to having administrative abilities. Furthermore, it is important that the director firmly believes that community-based work is an important component of client rehabilitation and that academic degrees do not determine the ability of follow-up paraprofessionals to carry out this work. It is helpful if the director is a medical doctor; this facilitates relationships with mental hospitals and expedites medication decisions. However, the most important competencies for the director are extensive training and experience in working with persons who have serious psychological difficulties, and an awareness of current research and service delivery developments.

Relationships with the Mental Health Center and State Hospital.   Staff members of the Cambridge-Somerville follow-up program believe that a good follow-up program should link the hospital to various center and community service programs while maintaining fiscal and administrative autonomy from the organizations with which it interacts. Such autonomy helps the program to focus its services on clients, rather than on the needs of mental health organizations.

At Cambridge-Somerville, the follow-up staff members also maintain that an effective follow-up program requires cooperation and services from various organizations. Staff members from the other center programs will be more likely to cooperate if their own representatives are involved in the initial planning of the follow-up program. Staff members from mental hospitals in the service area will be more helpful if the program director makes a point of spending some time at these hospitals, establishing relationships and mutual trust.

Services to Patients Prior to Discharge.   Ideally, a follow-up program initiates contact with its clients by providing predischarge services while the clients are still within a state or other long-term mental hospital. Such predischarge services are best provided within wards organized to correspond with center neighborhoods. If the hospital is located in the same community as the mental health center, the program paraprofessionals and other staff members should be careful not to compete with services already provided by the hospital social workers.

If the hospital is located at a considerable distance from the center, the program staff members may wish to train hospital employees to carry out predischarge planning. This training may prove a difficult task, since hospital employees are sometimes oriented toward retaining rather than discharging clients. Even when working with a distant hospital, it is desirabale for paraprofessional staff members to meet with patients prior to discharge. At the time of discharge, paraprofessionals can provide transportation back to their communities for patients who lack means of transportation.

Transferability to an Inpatient Program.   Many centers may wish to provide follow-up services to clients in the center's own inpatient ward. The follow-up paraprofessionals in the Cambridge-Somerville ACS program agreed that their services would be relevant to inpatient clients lacking family ties, disability insurance, and other basic resources for living. Because inpatient wards are typically short-term facilities, the follow-up discharge planning should be carried out quickly and efficiently. The follow-up services could be provided by a separate follow-up program, or the inpatient staff could be trained in follow-up functions. Community-based functions would add variety to the jobs of inpatient staff members, and demonstrate to them that nonclinical services can contribute to client progress. It would be necessary, however, to reassure discharged patients that the inpatient staff members would not utilize their community-based input to try to identify reasons for readmitting former patients. Furthermore, ward procedures would have to be restructured in order to provide community release time for inpatient staff members.

Follow-up by Geriatric and Alcoholism Programs.   At the Cambridge-Somerville center, the geriatric and alcohol-abusing clients are served by special follow-up teams. As an alternative, follow-up services to these types of clients could be provided by appropriately trained paraprofessionals from a center's geriatric and alcoholism services.

Possible Prevention Services by Follow-up Workers.   The community-based services that the Cambridge-Somerville workers are trained to provide are potentially useful to noninstitutionalized individuals who require assistance with housing, welfare, vocational rehabilitation, and daily living needs. In some cases these services could prevent the future institutionalization of seriously upset people who are experiencing difficulty in coping with the problems of everyday life.

A follow-up program can increase the impact of its prevention-oriented efforts by offering consultation and education services to staff members of relevant agencies and community organizations. For example, follow-up paraprofessionals could provide case consultation services designed to train welfare workers to recognize and refer clients who are unable to cope with daily living needs. The paraprofessionals could also, for example, train probation officers to instruct community volunteers in the skills required to help clients on probation with housing, welfare, and vocational rehabilitation placement. Training also could be offered to service personnel at Spanish-speaking community organizations to teach procedures for helping new Spanish-speaking residents to obtain housing and welfare.

Paraprofessionals in a Follow-up Program.   A follow-up paraprofessional must be able to work within a highly structured hospital setting as well as autonomously within the community. The specific skills required include the ability to establish trusting relationships with hospital and agency staff and with clients, work up discharge plans, handle unruly clients in hospital wards, and provide various follow-up services in community settings. Follow-up paraprofessionals should be carefully selected and then given extensive training and supervision as well as moral support.

Follow-up work requires considerable effort, a variety of skills, and the ability to tolerate repeated frustrations. Follow-up workers should receive salaries that adequately reflect the high demands of their work. In the absence of equitable salaries, a high staff turnover rate may reduce continuity of care and program cost-effectiveness.

After a follow-up program has been in operation for a time, staff members may wish to provide formal therapy services for their clients. This outcome follows logically as a consequence of program operations. As a hospital population is reduced through the deinstitutionalization program, follow-up workers may find that time has become available both for performing more specialized services for their clients and for learning new competencies. Follow-up clients may not be willing or able to go to an outpatient program. Likewise, outpatient staff members often prefer to deal with less disturbed and less chronic clients. The Cambridge-Somerville staff members believe that follow-up paraprofessionals can be effective as therapists if they receive appropriate training prior to providing therapy and receive ongoing weekly supervision from skilled clinicians.

Ideas for Implementing an Outpatient Program

The use of paraprofessionals to provide outpatient services allows a community mental health center to broaden substantially the number and range of these services. This is particularly true in terms of less traditional outpatient tasks that involve working in the community as opposed to working in an office.

Recruitment and Selection.   It is helpful if the paraprofessionals are from the same community and ethnic group as the client population they are to serve. Such commonality may establish useful ties between the center and the community. When selecting paraprofessionals to provide the types of services they do in the Orange County outpatient program, potential staff member's background of either paid or volunteer experience working with people in a helping capacity also is considered.

Training.   Training should be provided to build on the general knowledge and talents of the paraprofessionals. This should include not only an initial orientation, but an ongoing program designed to increase necessary skills. Ideally, this training should be accredited and in other ways linked to established educational programs at nearby colleges and universities. Energy and time spent in training should result not only in increased personal responsibilities, but also should be rewarded by increased status and salary.

Supervision.   To maintain a community-based task orientation in outpatient services, supervisors should hold a nontraditional outpatient service philosophy. In the Orange County model, such activities as in-community crisis work, client advocacy, social agency coordination, assisting clients to obtain available social services, assistance with employment seeking, program development with alternative agencies, and educational activities with schools are seen as tasks appropriate for outpatient staff, and closely related to the goal of improved mental health for clients.

Ideas for Implementing a Screening Program

The Roxbury Court Clinic, the program selected for a case study in the area of screening services, provides all federally required screening services for adult offenders. In addition, it provides a number of innovative features and interventions that are very unusual in screening programs. However, when considered in isolation from the mental health center with which it is affiliated, Roxbury Court Clinic does not offer the full array of screening services required by the 1975 federal community mental health legislation. More specifically, it does not serve children and adolescents, nor does it provide screening services (with the exception of walk-in clients who request services) for adults who have not been in contact with a court system. This section offers suggestions concerning the incorporation of the clinic's services into a full-scale screening program and the transferring of the Roxbury Court model to other community mental health centers.

The Roxbury Court Clinic can arrange treatment as an alternative to incarceration, both for offenders committed to inpatient facilities and for offenders who do not require inpatient treatment. However, as in most diversion programs, data have not been gathered proving that treatment, in and of itself, reduces recidivism among offenders who are not confined in treatment facilities. The assumption that reduced recidivism can be used as a measure of program success, furthermore, raises larger questions about the relationship between mental health problems and crime. Evidence from the Roxbury Clinic and other sources suggests that the broader social factors that contribute to recidivism cannot be completely counteracted solely by mental health treatment strategies.

Creating a Full-scale Screening Program. If a community mental health center simply wishes to comply with the minimal requirements of federal legislation, it can provide screening services at the mental health center for clients being considered for commitment to inpatient treatment programs. A centralized intake unit can employ staff members trained to diagnose mental health problems and formulate treatment plans for the normal and retarded children, adolescents, and adults referred for screening by courts, schools, and other agencies. However, a closer association with community agencies such as courts has many advantages, as demonstrated by the Roxbury Court Clinic.

Implementation of Screening within Agencies. The Roxbury Court Clinic provides a model for offering screening services within a community agency. Often working within the cellblock itself, the clinic's staff members screen individuals for whom inpatient commitment is being considered, as well as many other clients of the court who have mental problems but who otherwise might not seek or receive mental health services. As an added feature, a court clinic's staff members can provide expert consultation to the parent mental health center on cases where legal considerations are involved.

A program similar to the Roxbury Court Clinic could be established within a juvenile court. The program would differ from the Roxbury model in that the staff members would be trained to work with the problems of a juvenile population; to establish liaisons with schools, foster homes, and community programs for children and adolescents; and to work closely with parents. The schools or parents could be included in the implementation of treatment plans.

Transferring the Roxbury Court Model. The most readily transferable feature of the Roxbury model is the one-to-one screening service. Screening services provide the greatest benefit to the court and client if carried out on a pretrial basis. Once the court realizes the value of pretrial screening, its demands for screening services may become heavy. As a result, it may become impossible for a screening program to provide the Roxbury Clinic's other intervention services for clients or for its alcohol and drug screening programs unless funding and priorities for these additional services are firmly established.

The judge is the key person in the establishment of a court clinic. However, many judges do not perceive a connection between criminal behavior and mental and social conditions. Thus, one appropriate aspect of a screening program would be education of the judiciary concerning the benefits of a broader outlook. One possible result of such an effort could be judicial interest in effective rehabilitation services for clients. It is also important to cultivate similar ties with the probation department.

Sound working relationships should be established with the community-based drug and alcohol treatment agencies with which a court clinic collaborates. Such agencies can be induced to work with a clinic by offering them the possibility of referrals, for which the agencies receive third-party reimbursements. The outcome of treatment is probably determined largely by the quality of the treatment program to which the client is referred. It is therefore crucial for the clinic to refer its clients to reputable and competent treatment agencies. Ideally, a clinic would conduct routine, periodic follow-up checks on the progress of each of its clients, and occasionally would verify through site visits that the agencies are providing quality services and safeguarding the civil rights of clients.

The director of a court clinic should be skillful at building relationships with other organizations—the court, community-based treatment agencies, and the community mental health center. It is likely that the director will spend considerable time on various public commissions, in liaison work, and in promoting high morale among clinic staff. Administrative skills are, thus, at least as important as clinical skills in the choice of a clinic director.

Paraprofessionals in a Screening Program.   The screening of adult offenders requires a combination of interviewing and diagnostic skills. The diagnostic skills are probably best developed by involvement in a well-designed training program. Ideally, the paraprofessionals would be trained to devise a complete psychosocial work-up to be submitted to a professional who is an expert in implementing these procedures and interpreting the results. The interviewing skills involve training and an ability, often acquired prior to formal training, to be both easygoing and hard-hitting with individuals accused of moderate to serious crimes.

Paraprofessionals or professionals involved in screening should be closely supervised by professionals who themselves are trained in diagnostic techniques and in formulating diagnosis-based treatment plans. This supervision is especially important in cases where a client is being screened for commitment to an inpatient treatment facility. When any doubt arises in these cases, the supervising professional should take responsibility for carrying out the complete screening procedure. Most professionals, it should be noted, are probably not prepared by their graduate school training for effective implementation of court clinic screening and supervision procedures.

Judges who observe that paraprofessionals can perform with a high level of competence will probably become more open to accepting recommendations from these clinic staff members. Initially, professional-paraprofessional teams might jointly present recommendations to a judge. As the judge becomes more accustomed to listening to paraprofessionals, the paraprofessionals can begin to make recommendations on their own.

REFERENCE NOTE

1.   Alley, S. R., Blanton, J., & Feldman, R. E. (Eds.). *Paraprofessionals in mental health: Theory and practice.* Book in preparation, 1977.

REFERENCES

Larsen, J. K., & Norris, E. L. Consultation to mental health agencies: What makes it work (or not)? *Innovations,* 1977, *4*(2), 25–28.
Social Action Research Center. *Paraprofessionals in mental health: An annotated bibliography from 1966 to 1977.* Oakland, California: Diana Press, in press.

RESOURCES

This appendix contains further information that was gathered during our past year's research. This information could be of practical value to a mental health organization which is considering the use of paraprofessionals or seeking to improve the service delivery of their present staff members.

GENERAL REFERENCES ON PARAPROFESSIONALS

This section contains a list of books and articles with descriptive annotations that examine the use of paraprofessionals from various perspectives. Items are drawn from our bibliography, *Paraprofessionals in Mental Health: An Annotated Bibliography from 1966 to 1977.*

Albee, G. W.
Conceptual Models and Manpower Requirements in Psychology.
American Psychologist, 1968, *23*(5), 317–320.
Discusses the problem of the present and prospective shortage of professional mental health workers as deriving from the disease model of mental disorder; proposes that this model be abandoned and reconceptualized, and that alternatives be found; suggests that development of an institutional structure would enable the use of easily recruited and trained B.A.-level personnel.

Alley, S. R., Blanton, J., & Feldman, R. E. (Eds.)
Paraprofessionals in Mental Health: Theory and Practice.
New York: Human Sciences Press, 1979.

Contains 15 original chapters by national authorities on the use of paraprofessionals in mental health, covering these topics: (1) philosophy of paraprofessional use; (2) history of paraprofessionals; (3) paraprofessionals in a comprehensive community mental health center; (4) a system-wide program for use of paraprofessionals; (5) guidelines for the indigenous change agent; (6) a needs-based service delivery model; (7) evaluation of the effectiveness of paraprofessionals in service-delivery; (8) evaluation of paraprofessional programs; (9) achievement of economic efficiency with paraprofessionals; (10) training, supervision, and evaluation of paraprofessionals; (11) a human service generalist framework for integrating and utilizing all levels of staff; (12) promoting collaboration between professionals and paraprofessionals and between an urban community and its mental health center; (13) paraprofessionals in psychosocial community programs; (14) the new volunteer; and (15) self-help.

Arnhoff, F. N., Rubinstein, E. A., & Speisman, J. C.
Manpower for Mental Health.
Chicago: Aldine, 1969.
Based on the papers and proceedings of a symposium sponsored by the National Institute of Mental Health, entitled "Manpower and Mental Health," in Warenton, Virginia, 1967. The symposium examined specific concepts and theoretical issues of importance in mental health manpower policy and in the further development of the entire mental health program; also considers issues that have significance for total program implementation; how the composition, patterns, and trends of the total labor force complex relate to mental health manpower; and what changes will be needed in the future.

Berman, G. S., & Haug, M. R.
New Careers: Bridges or Ladders?
Social Work, 1973, *18*(4), 48–58.
Points out a conflict in two objectives of the paraprofessional model—to open pathways for upward mobility in service jobs and to use indigenous people as mediators between agency and clientele; investigates the extent to which this potential dilemma is reflected in the aspirations of paraprofessional trainees.

Blanton, J., & Alley, S. R.
Models of Program Success in New Careers Programs.
Journal of Community Psychology, in press.
Describes variables related to the successful achievement of goals of new careers programs; uses correlations, path analysis, and case study data to develop models of successful program functioning; results show that factors affecting programmatic success were: (1) the use of a system of program planning and self-assessment; (2) the ability of the staff to influence relevant outside agencies and groups informally; and (3) the employment of staff or consultants who have capacity in all critical areas. Indicates applicability to other human service projects.

Brown, B. S.
The Training of Mental Health Auxiliaries for Mental Health Care.
Paper presented at the Annual Meeting of the Indian Psychiatric Society in Trivandrum, India, January 1975.
Summarizes and describes the evolution of the mental health worker concept and the

New Careers Training Program; provides a brief historical overview of advances made in research on mental illness in the last few decades and of public mental health services in the U. S.; stresses the need for nations to collaborate on and share advances in the field; outlines public mental health service programs and the relationship between and role differentiation of professionals and paraprofessionals; emphasizes the need for preventive medicine and care on a worldwide basis.

Cohen, R.
"New Careers" Grows Older: A Perspective on the Paraprofessional Experience, 1965–1975.
Baltimore, Maryland: Johns Hopkins University Press, Policy Studies in Employment and Welfare, Number 26, 1976.
Summarizes the New Careers experience during the period from 1965 to 1975 and briefly describes the history and development of New Careers; delineates the goals of New Careers programs; includes statistical data about paraprofessionals and examples of New Careers functions and programs; overviews critical issues such as recruitment, training, supervision, and mobility. Concludes with assessment of the status and impact of the New Careers imovement and speculations about the future.

Dugger, J. G.
The New Professional: Introduction for the Human Services/Mental Health Worker.
Monterey, California: Cole Publishing, 1975.
Sketches the development of the new professional through the community mental health movement and the paraprofessional movement of the 1960s; also sketches Riessman's "helper-therapy" principle and the concept of the indigenous worker. Discusses topics on behavior differences, cultural differences, intervention techniques, crisis problems, group dynamics, group leadership, community resources, and working with data.

Durlak, J. A.
Myths Concerning the Nonprofessional Therapist.
Professional Psychology, 1973, *4*(3), 300–304.
Tries to dispel prominent myths, both negative and positive, concerning the nonprofessional therapist by basing conclusions on existing clinical evidence.

Gartner, A.
Paraprofessionals and Their Performance: A Survey of Education, Health, and Social Service Programs.
New York: Praeger Publishers, 1971.
Analyzes the research on the paraprofessional in a variety of fields: health, education, social service, corrections, and mental health. Presents a highly balanced picture of the accomplishments of paraprofessional workers; covers not only all the existing literature, but also develops important insights regarding a variety of issues: the relationship of indigeneity and training, the relationship of the paraprofessional and the professional, and the relationship of the paraprofessional and the community.

Gartner, A., & Riessman, F.
Changing the Professions: The New Careers Strategy.
In R. Gross & P. Osterman (Eds.), *The New Professionals.*
New York: Simon and Schuster, 1972.
Discusses the New Careers strategy which seeks to change professional practices, roles,

institutions, functions, values, and attitudes; points out that the paraprofessional improves both the efficiency and the productivity of the system by sensitizing professionals in the work place and, to a lesser extent, in the training process.

Grosser, C., Henry, W. E., & Kelly, J. G.
Nonprofessionals in the Human Services.
San Francisco: Jossey-Bass, 1969.
Covers the role of the paraprofessional in the mental health field and provides a working compendium for the layman in the community as well as for the professional; a joint effort made possible by the National Association of Social Workers and the American Psychological Association.

Guerney, B. G. (Ed.)
Psychotherapeutic Agents: New Roles for Nonprofessionals, Parents, and Teachers.
New York: Holt, Rinehart and Winston, 1969.
Presents historical developments and factual considerations which underlie the strategy of using nonprofessionals as therapeutic agents; also presents specifically, and in some detail, remedial methods and procedures based on this strategy.

Hines, L.
A Nonprofessional Discusses Her Role in Mental Health.
American Journal of Psychiatry, 1970, *126*(10), 1467–1472.
Describes the author's period of training as a mental health assistant and her current work with individual patients, home visiting, child and parent groups, and the homemaking service she is developing in the Temple University Community Mental Health Center. She concludes that although mental health centers cannot solve all of society's problems, they must expand their services to meet the needs of the total community, as well as its patients, if they are to be truly effective in the promotion of mental health.

Kalafat, J., & Boroto, D. R.
The Paraprofessional Movement as a Paradigm Community Psychology Endeavor.
Journal of Community Psychology, 1977, *5,* 3–12.
Asserts that community psychology can be seen as a vigorous, action-oriented movement, but still in the development state, and that the growing paraprofessional movement shares similar origins to community psychology and appears to provide answers to some of the questions raised about the accomplishments of the practitioners of community psychology; briefly reviews some of the stated goals of community psychology, and describes the paraprofessional movement in greater detail to demonstrate the relationship between the accomplishments and trends of the paraprofessional movement and the goals espoused by community psychologists.

Karlsruher, A. E.
The Nonprofessional as a Psychotherapeutic Agent: A Review of the Empirical Evidence Pertaining to His Effectiveness.
American Journal of Community Psychology, 1974, *2*(1), 61–77.
Examines the literature pertaining to the psychotherapeutic effectiveness of nonprofessionals: Reports empirical evidence that nonprofessionals can facilitate the improvement of psychotic adult inpatients but cannot effectively serve outpatient adults or adolescents and children at this time. The comparative effectiveness of nonprofessional

and professional psychotherapists has not been adequately examined, nor have the factors which contribute to the psychotherapeutic effectiveness of nonprofessionals. Since nonprofessionals are destined to provide a significant portion of therapeutic service, it is imperative that adequate investigations of their effectiveness be carried out.

Matarazzo, J. D.
Some National Developments in the Utilization of Nontraditional Mental Health Manpower.
American Psychologist, 1971, *26*(4), 363–372.
States that while the membership of the four traditional mental health professions (psychiatry, psychology, social service, nursing) continues even today to debate the need for and means of recruiting other types of personnel to help provide services to this country's mentally ill and emotionally disturbed, other segments of society have recruited, trained, and already put to work thousands of nonprofessional persons whose major qualification is a desire to help fellow human beings.

Pearl, A., & Riessman, F.
New Careers for the Poor: The Nonprofessional in Human Service.
New York: The Free Press, 1965.
A major source in guiding the formulation of New Careers policies, both in mental health and other disciplines. Contains chapters on specialized topics by a number of authorities; describes strategies for combining the provision of career opportunities for the poor with improved and more relevant services to consumers; combines discussions of specialized issues with coverage of general topics, such as education as a model for New Careers, issues and pitfalls in the New Careers movement, and New Careers' allies.

Riessman, F., & Popper, H. I.
Up from Poverty: New Career Ladders for Nonprofessionals.
New York: Harper & Row, 1968.
Examines the concepts underlying new careers as "an expression of faith in the ability of the more and the less privileged" to join in mutual goals and programs, and as a practical instrument of social change. Designed to be a handbook for those active in the field and a guidebook for those who are not; considers new careers from the point of view of the public and several societal institutions such as social welfare, the schools, health services, and corrections. Concludes with ideas for future policy.

Sobey, F.
The Nonprofessional Revolution in Mental Health.
New York: Columbia University Press, 1970.
Points out that nonprofessionals are utilized not simply because professional manpower is unavailable but rather to provide new services in innovative ways; states that nonprofessionals are being trained for new service functions and roles, some of which were not previously being played at all in the mental health program.

SERVICE SPECIFIC REFERENCES

This next section presents books and articles relevant to the use of paraprofessionals in specific mental health service areas. This list of references cannot be considered complete or definitive, but should give readers a place to begin in their search for information on various service areas. We have categorized the readings by service area.

Aging

Bowles, E.
Older Persons as Providers of Services: Three Federal Programs.
Social Policy, 1976, *7*(3), 81–88.
Contends that programs such as the Foster Grandparent Program (FGP), Senior Companion Program (SCP), and the Retired Senior Volunteer Program (RSVP) are a strong argument for further developing and utilizing the skills of the elderly. The paraprofessional functions performed by FGP, SCP, and RSVP volunteers demonstrate that many older persons are interested in and capable of utilizing new knowledge and skills.

Gray, R. M., & Kasteler, J. M.
An Evaluation of the Effectiveness of a Foster Grandparent Project.
Sociology and Social Research, 1970, *54*(2), 181–189.
Evaluates the effects of a foster grandparent project employing needy elderly to work with retarded children: Fifty-two elderly employees who had participated in the program for one year were chosen as the experimental group and compared to a nonparticipant elderly group (N = 52). The two groups did not differ significantly on pretest measures or demographic variables. Using the Your Attitudes and Activities inventory and the Neugarten Life Satisfaction Rating Scale, the experimental group was found to have benefited in the areas of personal and social adjustment and life satisfaction relative to the control subjects. No evaluation of benefits to the children is presented.

Hoff, W.
Training the Disadvantaged as Home Health Aides.
Public Health Reports, 1969, *84*, 617–623.
Describes a pilot training project (in Oakland, California) to test how effectively older unemployed men and women in poverty areas could be recruited and trained to provide nursing care for ill people in their homes; states that principles of programmed learning were followed to: (1) determine the characteristics of the trainees; (2) identify behavioral objectives; (3) break subject matter into small, discrete steps; (4) arrange learning in a progressive sequence; and (5) allow trainees to progress at their own speed. The results of this evaluation showed that all the aides were performing at or above satisfactory levels.

Lake, G.
The Training, Supervision, and Utilization of Geriatric Outreach Workers.
American Journal of Orthopsychiatry, 1972, *42*(2), 334–335.
Describes an ongoing experimental and demonstration training program which drew on inner-city people and many diverse agencies serving the elderly for the purpose of extending a new kind of assistance to the elderly; describes results as an improvement in their ability to function in their own homes, relief from some difficulties of daily living, and avoidance of institutionalization except for severe medical reasons; says that the program also serves as a catalyst in drawing together, as planners and teachers, agencies and individuals concerned with providing health and social services to the elderly in the community.

Patterson, R. D.
Services for the Aged in Community Mental Health Centers.
American Journal of Psychiatry, 1976, *133*(3), 271–273.
Studies services provided for the elderly at eight federally funded community mental health centers; describes discrimination against the elderly, the reasons why relatively few elderly persons seek care, and innovations in treatment. It was discovered that high-quality care depends more on staff awareness of the unique problems of the elderly than on specialized services. Recommends a more public health-oriented approach that would set priorities on the basis of community needs.

Rivesman, L.
Utilization of Paraprofessionals for Services to the Aged in Family Service Agencies.
American Journal of Orthopsychiatry, 1972, *42*(2), 341–342.
Summarizes the process and findings of a project aimed at the improvement of the quality of service to family agency clients aged 60 and over: Within the overall purpose of service enhancement, the use of paraprofessionals was tested through the development of service dyads consisting of a professional-educated caseworker (MSW) and an assistant of mature age (35 and over). The graduate practitioner was responsible for the training and supervision of her assistant as well as for the assignment of those "tasks" on her caseload that were deemed appropriate for the assistant.

Suffolk County Health Services, Community Mental Health Division.
Outreach for the Aged.
Hauppauge, New York: Author, 1976.
States that the Community Mental Health Division of the County Health Services Department has the responsibility for the planning and delivery of mental health services to area residents; says that this program recognizes the paucity of mental health services to the elderly of this community, and proposes to deal with this lack by training staff of senior centers in outreach and intervention skills; includes crisis intervention, problem solving, and referral skills.

Alcohol

Cooke, G., Whemer, G., & Gruber, J.
Training Paraprofessionals in the Treatment of Alcoholism: Effects on Knowledge, Attitudes and Therapeutic Techniques.
Quarterly Journal of Studies on Alcohol, 1975, *36*(7), 938–948.
Discusses an experiment in which participation in a paraprofessional training program increased the trainees' knowledge of alcoholism, modified their attitudes toward alcoholism, and affected their therapeutic techniques; gives data on time involved and type of curriculum for trainees; concludes that, in general, younger trainees with a higher education level, a more positive attitude toward need for treatment, greater initial knowledge, and higher scores on four personality scales gained more knowledge from the training program; concludes further that certain backgrounds and personality characteristics can be associated with differential gains from training.

Ferneau, E., & Paine, H. J.
Attitudes Regarding Alcoholism: The Volunteer Alcoholism Clinic Counselor.
British Journal of Addiction, 1972, *67*(4), 235–238.
Presents a study which administered the Alcoholism Questionnaire to 11 paraprofes-

sional trainees in alcoholism counseling at the beginning of an intensive 10-week training course; computes and compares nine mean factor scores to those of a norm group: Volunteer subjects were more likely (1) not to believe that the alcoholic comes from lower socioeconomic strata, (2) to believe that alcoholism is an illness, (3) to believe that the alcoholic is not just a harmless heavy drinker, and (4) to believe that alcohol is highly addictive. In addition, subjects were even less likely than the norm group to see the alcoholic as a weak-willed person.

Kalb, M., & Propper, M. S.
The Future of Alcohology: Craft or Science?
American Journal of Psychiatry, 1976, *133*(6), 641–645.
Discusses the problems resulting from the influx of professionals into the field of alcoholism which has historically been dominated by paraprofessional workers. The interaction of the professional alcohologist, who operates from a scientific model, with the paraprofessional worker, whose model of treatment has followed craft lines, has created unique problems and tensions. A synergism has been created which has been detrimental rather than complementary. Suggested that the future of the alcoholism field will have to be established along craft (paraprofessional) or scientific (professional) lines because the two models cannot profitably coexist.

Staub, G. E., & Kent, L. M. (Eds.)
Paraprofessional in the Treatment of Alcoholism: A New Profession.
Springfield, Illinois: Charles C Thomas, 1973.
Reviews and discusses the wide range of philosophies and policies related to the work of a paraprofessional in the field of alcoholism; covers such subjects as on-the-job training, differences between nonalcoholic and recovered alcoholic counselor personnel, and the roles of administrators and paraprofessionals operating within poverty communities, medical situations, and outpatient clinics. The contents are designed to assist individuals involved in program planning, personnel development, training, teaching, and interdisciplinary teamwork.

Teicher, J. D., Sinay, R., & Stumphauzer, J. S.
Training Community-Based Paraprofessionals as Behavior Therapists with Families of Alcohol-Abusing Adolescents.
American Journal of Psychiatry, 1976 *133*(7), 846–850.
Describes a pilot program which was established in California to train 10 paraprofessionals to conduct behavioral family therapy directly in the homes of alcohol-abusing adolescents. Trained as a group for six months, the paraprofessionals attended weekly didactic and workshop sessions. Each of the four paraprofessionals who completed training treated three families using behavioral contracting methods. Conclusions state that this program is a viable model for training paraprofessionals in this problem area and subsequently for community intervention for a wide variety of family problems.

Children

Cowen, E. L., Trost, M. A., & Izzo, L. D.
Nonprofessional Human-Service Personnel in Consulting Roles.
Community Mental Health Journal, 1973, *9*(4), 335–341.
Describes an experiment in which four nonprofessionals (housewives), each with six

years of prior experience as child aides in a school mental health program for early detection and prevention of school maladaptation, assumed consultative responsibilities in an expanded project involving 12 schools and 60 child aides. The nonprofessional consultants engaged in a variety of functions including aide serving, child serving, professional team serving, administrative, and research activities. Consultants were most effective, most satisfied, and contributed most to programs in roles that directly tapped their own prior school experiences, rather than when viewed simply as an "extra pair of hands."

Epstein, N., & Shainline, A.
Paraprofessional Parent-Aides and Disadvantaged Families.
Social Casework, 1974, *55*(4), 230–236.
Describes a one-year experimental program designed to provide a paraprofessional parent-aide service to chronic multiproblem families; establishes goals to offer in-home rehabilitation, counseling, and guidance service to families with problems in child rearing, to train adult paraprofessionals as parent-aides in family living and child rearing with expertise in working with families within their home settings, to test the feasibility of group meetings for sharing problems, and to offer an alternative to hospitalization. Seventeen families were served, with aides spending 65% of their time in direct contact and 20% devoted to telephone contacts. Parents reported marked differences in their living situations as a result of the help provided by the parent-aides.

Fishman, J., Mitchell, L. E., & Wittenberg, C.
Baker's Dozen: A Program of Training Young People as Mental Health Aides.
Mental Health Program Reports, 1968, *2,* 11–24.
Reports on Baker's Dozen (affiliated with the Institute for Youth Studies at Howard University)—a mental health aide training program for indigenous youth who reside in a poverty area in Washington, D.C., to provide mental health service to one or more groups of disturbed, needy adolescents. States that the help provided by the trainees is given at less cost and more effectively than it could be given by a program limited to traditional use of professionals. Discusses characteristics of the area, and the issues of recruitment and selection; training is discussed in depth. Concludes with discussion of other issues such as: the differing backgrounds and attitudes of professional staff and the mental health aides, the needs of paraprofessionals, and job mobility.

Gardner, J. E.
Paraprofessionals Work with Troubled Children.
New York: Gardner Press, 1975.
Reports on and describes the various projects which have been developed and maintained to make extensive use of paraprofessionals at the Children's Center for Educational Therapy in Venice, California; intends to stimulate the development and/or amplification of such programs in other communities, agencies, clinics, and organizations.

Goodman, G.
Companionship Therapy.
San Francisco: Jossey-Bass, 1972.
Describes an experiment with nonprofessional therapists in a community setting which

studied the structure, process, and effects of therapies using nonprofessional or para-professional agents with troubled elementary schoolboys as patients; reviews changes in the mental health field and outlines the scope and logic of nonprofessional therapy; presents in detail the Group Assessment of Interpersonal Traits (GAIT) along with findings on students' motives for participating in the nonprofessional therapist role; discusses the dimension and patterns of companionships as well as strategies for identifying characteristics of successful companionships; summarizes all findings, offers conclusions, recommends procedures for nonprofessional therapy projects, and speculates on new directions in the field. Organized as a manual for establishing and studying nonprofessional therapy projects.

Rieger, N. I., & Devries, A. G.
The Child Mental Health Specialist: A New Profession.
American Journal of Orthopsychiatry, 1974, *44*(1), 150–158.
Advocates the belief that effective treatment of emotionally disturbed and delinquent children requires not large number of specialists for special needs, such as child psychologists, child psychiatrists, special education teachers, etc. but generalists for the general needs of these children—young people who have received broad training in the different treatment needs of the various facilities dealing with emotionally disturbed or delinquent children and adolescents. Talented trainees can be selected from among high school graduates, junior college graduates, and from among college and postcollege graduates. This paper describes a specific training program for Child Mental Health Specialists at the Camarillo Children's Treatment Center in collaboration with a nearby college and junior college.

Shortinghuis, N. E., & Frohman, A.
A Comparison of Paraprofessional and Professional Success with Pre-school Children.
Journal of Learning Disabilities, 1974, *7*(4), 62–64.
Describes a study in which 21 children and their parents were served by paraprofessionals, and 16 children were served by professionals in the Portage Project—a home approach to the early education of handicapped children in a rural area. The Portage Project, using a precision teaching model, offered an opportunity to compare gains made by children when they were served by a paraprofessional or a professional. The results indicate that in this project, paraprofessionals were as effective in teaching specific behaviors as professionals.

Consultation and Education

Guerney, B. G.
Relationship Enhancement: Skill-Training Programs for Therapy, Problem Prevention, and Enrichment.
San Francisco: Jossey-Bass, 1977.
Presents Relationship Enhancement (RE) therapy for enriching personal relationships and preventing problems; although a training method in the use of specific psychological skills, emphasizes education in harmonious and nondestructive concepts and behavior skills to solve family conflicts; encompasses the principles of both relationship therapy and behavior modification for preventing and treating personal and interpersonal problems; includes the scientific studies which led to the development of the RE

method. Points to the potential for self-help programs by training former participant nonprofessionals as group or assistant group leaders in this method.

Keeley, S. M., Shemberg, K. M., & Ferber, H.
The Training and Use of Undergraduates as Behavior Analysts in the Consultative Process.
Professional Psychology, 1973, *4*(1), 59–63.
Describes a newly instituted, behaviorally oriented training program for subprofessionals—a 20-week behavior analyst training course developed in the psychology department with academic credit for undergraduates. Undergraduates, selected by grades and interviews, are trained in behavioral observation and consulting with agents of change in the community, primarily parents and teachers. Concludes that undergraduates functioning as behavior analysts in mental health centers, state hospitals, and school systems represent a relevant approach to meeting the manpower crisis in the delivery of clinical services.

Mann, P. A.
Student Consultants: Evaluations by Consultees.
American Journal of Community Psychology, 1973, *1,* 182–193.
Describes a mental health consultation program in which elementary schoolteachers in five schools participated. All teachers, both users and nonusers of the program, were asked to evaluate it by means of a questionnaire. A comparison of questionnaire responses by 25 users and 25 nonusers of consultation indicated that: (1) less experienced teachers of the upper three grades used consultation more often and more experienced teachers of lower grades used consultation less often than did teachers in the remaining two combinations of experience and grade level; (2) teachers using consultation gave more specific definitions of the consultant's function than did nonusers; (3) teacher-consultees who rated consultation high in usefulness reported that the consultant's behavior was in line with their expectations more often than did teacher-consultees who gave low ratings; (4) high raters also perceived more changes in children's behavior or their perceptions of children. Implications for consultation training and practice are discussed.

Signell, K. A.
Training Nonprofessionals as Community Instructors; Mental Health Education Model of Primary Prevention.
Journal of Community Psychology, 1975, *3*(4), 365–373.
Describes processes useful in training nonprofessionals to do mental health education work in the community; focuses on training parents from the community to instruct other parents in parent-child communication courses. An intensive training course builds confidence and group cohesion through role modeling and practice teaching experience. Stresses key principles in any such training program for nonprofessionals: respect for the feelings of trainees; acknowledgment of the relevance of their own life experiences to the work they are being trained for; and an emphasis on working in pairs to provide mutual support and feedback.

Signell, K. A.
On a Shoestring: A Consumer-Based Source of Personpower for Mental Health Education.
Community Mental Health Journal, 1976, *12*(4), 342–354.

Outlines a program for promoting mental health in the population by "giving away our skills" as mental health professionals; states that this kind of program can be started on a shoestring by a community mental health center, family service agency, or adult education program, consisting of teaching parent-child communication courses, until a network of nonprofessionals is established; explores strategies of setting up programs and shifting roles of the professionals toward the nonprofessionals; and presents research on the program's effectiveness with parents and the impact on the lives and self-images of the nonprofessional instructors themselves.

Suinn, R. M.
Training Undergraduate Students as Community Behavior Modification Consultants.
Journal of Counseling Psychology, 1974, *21*(1), 71–77.
Outlines a training program in behavior modification consultation; describes how undergraduates with little or no background in psychology were trained in behavioral interviewing and operant behavior modification program design. Discussion includes the screening, training procedures, and the effects achieved in actual consultation by the trainees.

Drugs

Baldwin, B., Liptzin, M., & Goldstein, B.
Youth Services: A Multi-faceted Community Approach to Drug Abuse.
Hospital and Community Psychiatry, 1973, *24*(10), 695–697.
Reports on the evolution of the 1960s drug crisis drop-in centers and hot lines into multiservice centers dealing with other problems of youth; describes such a center in Chapel Hill, North Carolina, which has established two programs—a residential center for heroin addicts and a foster home for runaways. Peer counselors in the facilities have proved valuable in helping disturbed youths.

Cutler, R.
Consultation and Training Project for Paraprofessional Drug Workers.
Conference paper presented at North America Congress on Alcohol and Drug Problems. Washington, D. C.: Alcohol and Drug Problems Association of North America, 1974.
Analyzes the operation and effectiveness of the National Institute of Drug Abuse-funded consultation and training project for paraprofessional drug workers at Montefiore Hospital and Medical Center in the Bronx, New York; discusses background issues related to development of the clinical training model and summarizes the two-stage implemental process—the needs assessment phase and the introductory training work emerging from needs assessment workups; cites staff limitations in a number of skill areas and positive results of initial clinical case seminars; discusses improved staff attitudes, attributed to the testing and implementation of newly acquired knowledge and techniques.

Dalali, I. D., Charuvastra, V., & Schlesinger, J.
Training of Paraprofessionals: Some Caveats.
Journal of Drug Education, 1976, *6*(2), 105–112.
Discusses some of the dynamics inherent in the training process involving exaddict

paraprofessional counselors; focuses on the threat to self-esteem implied in the training process for exaddict counselors; emphasizes the need for training such counselors thoughtfully; discusses the more successful techniques employed to insure sensitivity and effectiveness.

Deitch, D.
The End of the Beginning: Dilemmas of the Paraprofessional in Current Drug Abuse Treatment.
Unpublished manuscript, 1974. (Available from Social Action Research Center, Berkeley, California).
Attempts to dispel certain positive myths concerning the use of paraprofessionals in drug abuse treatment—points to weaknesses in their use; recognizes their exploitation; discusses dilemmas of paraprofessionals in residential treatment and outpatient settings. However, supports the validity of those paraprofessionals who have maintained upper-level positions.

Roessler, R., Cook, D., Salley, K., Griffen, P., & Hale, K.
Drug Dependence and Its Treatment.
JSAS *Catalog of Selected Documents in Psychology,* 1976.
Presents an annotated bibliography which attempts to draw together, in one source, recent information on treatment and rehabilitation of drug abusers; places special emphasis on annotating articles from 1970 to mid-1974; presents research studies in terms of purpose, sample, method, results, and conclusions; abstracts descriptive articles in a paragraph format. Material in the bibliography introduces the reader to a representative sample of the work done in drug rehabilitation during the early to mid-1970s; includes such topics as drug treatment, drug abuse prevention, drug addicts, treatment of drug abuse, and follow-up studies.

Sloan, J. L., & Lipscomb, W. R. A.
A Nonobtrusive Interview Technique for Drug Abuse Program Follow-up.
Community Mental Health Journal, 1975, *11*(4), 368 370.
Describes a study of former drug abuse program clients which employed paraprofessional streetworkers, indigenous to the area, as data gatherers, using an interview designed to appear to be casual conversation. Interviewers were trained in the use of a mnemonic device which allowed them to guide the conversation over 46 items of factual information.

Emergency

Farberow, N. L.
Training in Suicide Prevention for Professional and Community Agents.
American Journal of Psychiatry, 1969, *125*(12), 1702–1705.
The Los Angeles Suicide Prevention Center has been training mental health professionals, semiprofessionals (primarily graduate students in mental health disciplines), nonprofessional volunteers, and various community groups for about a decade. Describes the various types of training offered at the Los Angeles Suicide Prevention Center, and notes that a primary objective for both public and professionals is to diminish the taboo aspects of suicide.

Helig, S. M., Farberow, N. L., Litman, R. E., & Schneidman, E. S.
The Role of Nonprofessional Volunteers in a Suicide Prevention Center.
Community Mental Health Journal, 1968, *4*(4), 287–295.
Describes the procedures in the selection, training, and supervision of 10 nonprofessional volunteers to provide direct therapeutic crisis services to patients in a suicide prevention center. One year's experience indicates a high degree of proficiency achieved by the volunteer in the handling of suicidal crises. The volunteers' reactions to the program are reported. Significant problems for the agency emerged in reference to precipitous increase in size of staff communication and, for the volunteer, in stimulation of problems of identity and self-concept. The comments are limited to agency situations involving the use of nonprofessional volunteers in regular collaboration with a professional staff. Other models, such as entirely volunteer staffed groups, must be evaluated separately.

Nelson, R. H.
The Crisis Call Center and Its Volunteers: A Comparison of Views with Mental Health Professionals.
Journal of Community Psychology, 1974, *2*(3), 237–241.
Describes a study which tried to compare how different mental health workers in the agency network of a community perceived a Crisis Call Center (CCC) in that community. Distance scores between concepts on the Semantic Differential were used to determine how close mental health professionals and CCC volunteers perceived the CCC to be to the other mental health-related agencies in the community. This study also tried to determine which mental health related occupations the volunteers identified with. It was found that the volunteers tended to identify with all the occupational concepts that were used, but to different degrees. It was also found that the mental health professionals included the CCC in their cluster of helping agencies. Implications of those findings are discussed toward an increased understanding of the role of volunteers in community crisis efforts and of the interrelationships among service agencies.

Pretzel, P. W.
The Volunteer Clinical Worker at the Suicide Prevention Center.
Bulletin of Suicidology, 1970, (6), 29–34.
Discusses the use of nonprofessional volunteers in short-term crisis intervention techniques; describes the experience of the Los Angeles Suicide Prevention Center with nonprofessional volunteers. The average volunteer was a middle-aged, prosperous, stable, married woman with children, who had experienced some form of mental illness in her own family. Training included: (1) a four-week program meeting two full days a week with a 40-hour clinical practicum; (2) practice in handling telephone calls with close supervision; and (3) continued weekly meetings with case conferences. Stringent selection of volunteers and sensitivity to their morale (i.e., avoiding boredom) are stressed.

Follow-up

Alternatives to Inpatient Care: Keeping It Close to Home.
Innovations, 1973, *1*(1), 12–16.
Describes a community effort in crisis therapy aimed at replacing inpatient care in state institutions. Therapeutic teams of psychiatrists, psychologists, social workers, nurses,

occupational therapists, and psychiatric technicians work with patients in a given geographical area providing local inpatient, outpatient, and aftercare services as well as school and agency consultation and prevention services.

Bodie, M. K., & Sandiford, C. A.
Mental Health Associates: One Answer to the Manpower Shortage.
American Journal of Nursing, 1971, *71,* 1395–1396.
Reports on a program at the Georgia Mental Institute in Atlanta prompted by a shortage of professional psychiatric nurses. States that the two main objectives of the program are: (1) to hire college graduates as high-caliber auxiliary personnel to aid nursing staffs in providing therapeutic care to patients; and (2) to provide good in-service education programs for both the new workers ("mental health associates") and registered nurses working with psychiatric patients.

Ellsworth, R. B.
The Background of the Fort Meade Aide-Role Project.
In *Nonprofessionals in Psychiatric Rehabilitation.*
New York: Appleton-Century-Crofts, 1968.
A description of the Fort Meade Veterans Hospital Aide-Role Project, as well as the questions which led to its implementation, and a study (Ellsworth, Bryand, and Butler) which reported observations of the day-to-day interaction of the psychiatric aide and the patient. Findings, indicating that many of the behavioral changes in the patient rose out of the aide-patient interaction, led to this 1968 study with its goal of radically modifying the aide's role with respect to all phases of rehabilitation, including treatment and release planning.

Inpatient

Goldstein, K. M., & Blackman, S.
The Functioning of Technicians of an Inpatient Unit of a Community Mental Health Center.
Journal of Community Psychology, 1973, *1*(1), 16–17.
Studies the sources of conflict between nurses and nursing technicians on the inpatient unit of a community mental health center; reports data obtained from nurses, technicians, and other staff on the unit that indicated general agreement on the low status of the technician position. However, technicians had social exchange relationships (liking and helping) similar to those of nurses and were seen as functioning as well in their positions as were nurses in theirs.

Mynatt, C. F., & Bailey, A.
Patients Employed as Aide Assistants.
Hospital and Community Psychiatry, 1972, *23*(1), 7.
Reports on an experimental program in which psychiatric hospital patients, who have been unsuccessfully involved in traditional treatment programs, are employed as aide assistants in understaffed wards after participating in a four-week training period. States that the program has improved employee morale and provided a realistic basis for positive interaction between staff and patient, and that the patient-aide, in many instances, relates more empathetically to patients than the staff does. Such recognizably

productive activity has encouraged patient initiative and self-esteem and a successful discharge of 34 of 57 participants.

Peckham, R. A.
Role of the Indigenous Aide in the Rehabilitation Process.
Studies in Rehabilitation Counselor Training, 1969, *7,* 49–53.
Discusses the use of rehabilitation aides in an inner-city environment— "Detroit's Harlem." A model is presented where the indigenous counselors work within a single neighborhood block, gathering groups of five. The counselor carries the "cluster of five" from referral to completion and then begins the next cluster as a new case load of five. The effective use of the aide as a communicant at referral and also as a communicating participant throughout, serving as a block captain, does much to help solve the problems of "the inner-city client who carries a ton of misery on his back."

Poser, E. G.
The Effect of Therapists' Training on Group Therapeutic Outcome.
Journal of Consulting Psychology, 1966, *30*(4), 283–289.
Assesses the comparative efficacy of trained and untrained therapists (the untrained group was composed of undergraduate students) in group therapy for psychotic patients; measures outcome of therapy by changes in psychological test performances of 195 patients before and after five months of group therapy. Findings show that lay therapists (when a comparison was made with an untreated control group) achieved slightly better results than psychiatrists and psychiatric social workers doing group therapy with similar patients.

Willard, C.
Psychiatric Aides as Case Managers.
Hospital and Community Psychiatry, 1970, *21*(3), 93.
Describes the development of a program using ward aides as case managers in the psychiatric team of an acute intensive treatment unit; concludes that a stable personnel force and professional staff members who are receptive to the statements of the case managers are essential to the success of such a program.

Outpatient

Cudaback, D.
Case-Sharing in the AFDC Program: The Use of Welfare-Service Aides.
Social Work, 1969, *14* (3), 93–99.
Describes a project in which Aid to Families with Dependent Children (AFDC) mothers in a large urban California county were trained to assist welfare department line workers on a team basis. The aides' success in providing counseling and client services points the way toward new methods of improving social services for the disadvantaged.

Epstein, N., & Shainline, A.
Paraprofessional Parent-Aides and Disadvantaged Families.
Social Casework, 1974, *55*(4), 230–236.
Describes a one-year experimental program designed to provide a paraprofessional parent aide service to chronic multiproblem families; establishes goals to offer in-home rehabilitation, counseling, and guidance service to families with problems in child

rearing; to train adult paraprofessionals as parent aides in family living and child rearing with expertise in working with families within their home settings; to test the feasibility of group meetings for sharing problems; and to offer an alternative to hospitalization. Seventeen families were served, with aides spending 65% of their time in direct contact and 20% devoted to telephone contacts. Parents reported marked differences in their living situations as a result of the help provided by the parent aides.

Felton, G. S., Wallach, H. F., & Gallo, C. L.
Training Mental Health Workers to Better Meet Patient Needs.
Hospital and Community Psychiatry, 1974, *25*(5), 299–302.
Discusses a hospital-based training program for paraprofessional mental health workers which focuses on maximizing their human relations skills and providing continuous care to the patients from admission through discharge and readjustment to the community; states that in coordinated clinical, academic, and community experiences the trainee learns to act as a patient advocate, long-term therapist, and treatment integrator; details the training curriculum as both theory and application of group process and systems change as well as work in nonconventional community service agencies.

Hallowitz, E., & Riessman, F.
The Role of the Indigenous Nonprofessional in a Community Mental Health Neighborhood Service Center Program.
American Journal of Orthopsychiatry, 1967, *37*(4), 766–778.
Discusses methods for utilizing the particular styles and skills of indigenous nonprofessionals in a Neighborhood Service Center Program, delineates the role of the worker as a neighborhood friend rather than as a junior caseworker or junior community organizer; presents some issues and problems in the use and development of nonprofessionals.

Persons, R. W., Clark, C., Persons, M., Kadish, M., & Patterson, W.
Training and Employing Undergraduates as Therapists in a College Counseling Service.
Professional Psychology, 1973, *4*(2), 170–178.
Describes an innovative program for developing selected undergraduate students into functioning psychotherapists at Antioch College's Counseling Center and in other settings; states that their student therapists have done individual and group therapy, handled emergencies, taught courses, and served as consultants.

Transitional Care

Handschu, S. S.
Profile of the Nurse's Aide: Expanding Her Role as Psycho-social Companion to the Nursing Home Resident.
Gerontologist, 1973, *13*(3, Pt. 1), 315–317.
Reports results of interviews with 206 nurses' aides, working in nursing homes, which show that most are paid less than $80 per week and that only two-thirds receive any on-the-job training. Author suggests that the role of the nurse's aide be considered in overall planning in nursing homes.

Sandall, H., Hawley, T. T., & Gordon, G. C.
The St. Louis Community Homes Program: Graduated Support for Long-term Care.

American Journal of Psychiatry, 1975, *132*(6), 617–622.
Describes a group home program that has been operating successfully for three years in St. Louis, Missouri; program offers ex-mental hospital patients the opportunity to gradually acquire experience in living independently in the community by sharing an apartment with a group of patients; program demonstrates that long-term chronic patients can use this alternative, community living environment "as a springboard to personal growth and eventual autonomy."

JOURNALS

The following are commonly available journals that may contain articles that are relevent to the use of paraprofessionals in mental health.

American Journal of Community Psychology
American Journal of Orthopsychiatry
American Psychologist
Community Mental Health Journal
Counselor Education and Supervision
Evaluation
Hospital and Community Psychiatry
Innovations
Journal of Community Psychology

Journal of Counseling Psychology
Mental Hygiene
Personnel and Guidance Journal
Professional Psychology
Public Health Reports
Public Welfare
Rehabilitation Counseling Bulletin
Social Casework
Social Work

TELEPHONE SURVEY: CENTERS

A significant amount of time was spent during our original selection process in interviewing mental health center administrators by telephone. We were told about many programs that made excellent use of paraprofessionals in mental health service delivery. We were able, of course, to select only one program in each service area.

What follows in this section is a listing, by service area, of some of the centers and programs that were recommended to us as effective but which were not site visited. These programs reported using paraprofessionals in providing both traditional and innovative services. We felt that persons reading this book might find centers in their locale to be useful resources. We were able to use the notes from telephone interviews to provide brief descriptions of the programs, or to note selected features.

Alcohol Programs

Cambridge-Somerville Mental Health and Retardation Center
12 Maple Avenue
Cambridge, Massachusetts 02139
A multidisciplinary staff, including paraprofessional alcohol counselors, provides walk-in emergency services, outpatient services, consultation and education services, community residences, and a detoxification unit for persons with alcohol problems. In addition, outreach work is undertaken which includes case finding and education efforts.

Kaliki-Palana Alcohol Program
1700 Lanakila Avenue
Honolulu, Hawaii 96817

A single-state agency, this program coordinates various relevant organizations in a unified effort to work with persons having problems with alcohol. A National Institute of Alcoholism and Alcohol Abuse special grant allows for training of paraprofessionals working in these organizations.

North Central Florida Community Mental Health Center, Inc.
3615 S.W. 13th Street
Gainesville, Florida 32608

This center uses paraprofessionals to provide a wide variety of outreach-oriented alcohol services to a 10-county area. Staff members live in the community they service, and citizens' groups act in an advisory capacity. The center has developed career ladders based on a combination of education and experience. It provides funds for career development and has arranged for tuition waivers at a nearby university for its paraprofessional staff.

San Luis Valley Comprehensive Mental Health Center
1015 4th Street
Alamosa, Colorado 81101

Paraprofessionals provide outpatient, detoxification, day treatment, and related services as well as an outreach approach to persons with alcohol problems. The center provides organizational support to paraprofessionals in terms of weekly professional supervision, in-house training that is accredited through the state university, and paraprofessional involvement in staff selection.

West Central Community Services Center
1125 6th St. S.E.
Willmar, Minnesota 56201

This center coordinates an extensive eight-county multidisciplinary effort to help persons with alcohol problems. The program is accredited, responsible to a community-run substance abuse advisory board, and pays special attention to the proper training, education, and use of paraprofessionals.

Women's Rehabilitation Association
181 Second Avenue, Suite 200
San Mateo, California 94401

A predominantly paraprofessional staff develops and provides individual treatment programs for each client and will use any approach that will assist in the recovery process. Emphasis is placed on group therapy comprised of peer groups.

Children's Services

Kedren Community Mental Health Center
7760 South Central Avenue
Los Angeles, California 90001

A training program for "Child and Parent" paraprofessional workers is offered through the center. During the nine-month period of intensive training the trainees receive a $2.50 hourly wage, compensation for child care expenses, and academic credit toward a B.A. degree. Topics covered by the program include: behavior therapy services, psychoeducational services, counseling services, and social services. These services are oriented toward preschool and elementary school children with behavioral and learning problems and toward the families of these children. The training includes classroom learning of concepts, simulated application of principles, and supervised application of the intervention techniques. For information, write:

> Child-Parent Community Mental Health Worker Training Program
> 8803 South Broadway
> Los Angeles, California   90023

Prairie View Mental Health Center
P.O. Box 467
Newton, Kansas 67114

Paraprofessionals teach behavior management skills to schoolteachers and give prevention-oriented workshops on childrearing practices to parents of young children.

Salt Lake Community Mental Health Center
807 East South Temple
Salt Lake City, Utah 84102

Paraprofessionals are treatment agents in a behavior modification day care program for multiproblem, severely handicapped children.

Tucson Southern Counties Mental Health Services, Inc.
1935 South Sixth Avenue
P.O. Box 5481
Tucson, Arizona 85703

After consulting with school staff members, paraprofessionals observe "problem" children in school settings. Then the paraprofessionals present their observations at a case conference, where a treatment plan is jointly constructed by mental health center and school staff members.

Washtenaw County Community Mental Health Center
2929 Plymouth Road
Ann Arbor, Michigan 48105

Paraprofessionals staff a drop-in center located in a neighborhood where children are at a high risk for developing mental disorders. While visiting the center to accompany or drop off their children, parents can learn about child development issues.

Consultation and Education Services

Albert Einstein Community Mental Health and Mental Retardation Center
York and Tabor Roads
Philadelphia, Pennsylvania 19141

a.   A community listening post allows consultation and education paraprofessionals to talk to people from the community and to put these people into contact with appropriate resources. These resources include other citizens, grass roots organizations, public agencies, and the mental health center.

b.   A paraprofessional directs a support service for prevention programs in the catchment district. For example, the program consults with relevant community agencies, helps the agencies to raise funds, and puts agencies with similar interests in touch with one another.

Community Organization for Mental Health and Retardation, Inc.
107 E. Lehigh Avenue
Philadelphia, Pennsylvania 19125
Each year the paraprofessionals rotate to a new service area unit within the community mental health center. Furthermore, all the paraprofessionals employed by the center meet monthly to maintain communication with one another.

Hahnemann Community Mental Health Center
314 North Broad Street
Philadelphia, Pennsylvania 19102
a.   The program is concerned with offering services to high risk groups. For example, paraprofessionals meet with selected mothers in maternity wards to teach parenting skills; a paraprofessional who is a former heorin addict helps methadone clinic clients to strengthen their roles as parents; and paraprofessionals train special education teachers to offer a social problem-solving course to children. The "script" for this course (as well as a similar script for use by parents) can be obtained by writing Dr. Myrna Shure at the Hahnemann Center.
The program holds luncheons attended by community citizens and by representatives of both public and grass roots community organizations. At this forum the needs of the catchment area are assessed and the value of various consultation and education programs is discussed.

Lane County Community Mental Health Center
1857 University Street
Eugene, Oregon 97403
The center has received a two-year National Institute of Mental Health grant to train paraprofessionals in primary prevention outreach skills. The workers are learning skills on three levels: interpersonal skills, group leadership and facilitation skills, and community/institutional development.

Rockland County Community Mental Health Center
Sanatorium Road
Pomona, New York 10970
a.   A paraprofessional trains police officers in mental health skills.
b.   A paraprofessional coordinates a mental health consumer advocacy service that receives complaints from consumers and from professionals in the catchment district. After receiving the complaints, the service attempts to bring about a resolution of the underlying conflicts.

South Hills Health System Community Mental Health/Mental Retardation Center
1800 West Street
Homestead, Pennsylvania 15120
The program used a National Institute of Mental Health grant to identify children at high risk for school failure (grades K through 3) and to consult with school personnel

on appropriate interventions. Other procedures included: evaluation, preventive interventions directly with identified children, and intervention with parents and with the school and community as systems.

Wyandotte County Mental Health and Guidance Center, Inc.
Eaton at 36th Avenue
Kansas City, Kansas 66103

The program is developing a "Youth Self-Advocacy" service. Adult paraprofessionals meet with adolescents in formal and informal settings to establish ties. The paraprofessionals help the adolescents to identify their needs, devise strategies for getting these needs filled, and evaluate the eventual effect of their action strategies. The emphasis of the program is on enhancing the self-help competencies of youth, rather than on increasing the responsiveness of the agencies that the youth contact for support. With upper elementary school youth, the consultants teach their consultation skills to personnel who are in direct contact with this younger population.

Day Care Services

Granite Community Mental Health Center
156 Westminster Avenue
Salt Lake City, Utah 84115

Selected primarily from a Spanish-speaking community and possessing less than B.A. degrees, the paraprofessional staff members work in four areas: aftercare, day treatment, evening groups, and outreach. The services are affiliated with a Spanish-speaking task force from the catchment area community.

The day care unit of the mental health center is also a base for a Minority Human Service Training Program. The purpose of this program is to train people from minority and disadvantaged groups to provide mental health services to a population that is, for the most part, unreached by mental health services. The trainees achieve a two-year associate degree as Human Service Workers, with 90 university credit hours. They become competent practitioners in working in their own neighborhoods and in their own languages. The trainees receive training in interviewing techniques, crisis intervention, family and group counseling, all of which originate from learning how to formulate a case and establish a plan of action. They learn how to provide social services, from "hard" services (such as helping clients get on welfare, Social Security, or obtain food stamps), to counseling services—including visiting the individuals in their homes, their communities, or inpatient settings.

The Minority Human Service Training Program is an effort initiated, promoted, and led by the Salt Lake Spanish-Speaking Health and Mental Health Task Force and the Granite Community Mental Health Center. It is financially supported by the National Institute of Mental Health by a grant awarded to the Task Force.

Salt Lake Community Mental Health Center
807 East South Temple
Salt Lake City, Utah 84102

A paraprofessional directs a day-treatment program comprised of two components. One component is a structured, goal-oriented day program designed to help an individual function at the maximum practical level of independence. The program is designed to provide an orderly transition from hospital to community life. Activities provided include group and individual therapy, training in skills of basic living, and various social and recreational activities. Participants capable of job training and placement are referred to vocational rehabilitation, and their community therapeutic program is designed to provide support and direction toward the goal of employment. If the participant is not yet able to work, referral may be made to the second component of the program.

This program is directed toward meeting the recreational and day treatment needs of emotionally disturbed individuals whose potential for employment in the immediate future is low. It provides a variety of group recreational activities, and sponsors community activities, also supporting an active patient government program. While clients may progress from the program to employment, the program is set up to avoid placing unrealistically high demands on a client.

Tri-County Community Mental Health Center
2900 Hospital Drive
North Kansas City, Missouri 64115

An initial diagnosis is made by a staff member on the day that a new client is admitted; at the same time a treatment plan is formulated in consultation with the given client. Clients maintain a record of their individual treatment goals, and each day at a group meeting solicit from their peers ideas on relevant goals. Paraprofessionals are involved in these features of the program.

Tufts Community Mental Health Center
171 Harrison Avenue
Boston, Massachusetts 02111

Community meetings are held bi-weekly. Two times a year, a day is set aside for presentations to clients by the staff members of major program changes for implementation.

Emergency Services

Hahnemann Community Mental Health Center
314 North Broad Street
Philadelphia, Pennsylvania 19102

In this center paraprofessionals perform intake evaluations on homeless people who temporarily reside in the downtown area and who have been referred to the center's emergency services. The paraprofessionals have a broad knowledge of community resources which they use in referring clients to appropriate services within the catchment area. A number of clients are referred to the center by hospitals who are treating them for accidental injuries and other medical problems. Therefore the paraprofessional staff work with medical personnel. Professional staff, including psychiatrists, work in a team with paraprofessional personnel in the delivery of these emergency services.

Rockland Community Health Center
Sanatorium Road
Pomona, New York 10970

This center uses a crisis telephone counseling service called "Open line." It is a county-wide information or referral crisis telephone service. It is staffed by paraprofessional personnel and 20 volunteers. Open line personnel provide crisis counseling on a range of problems from teenage romances to marital conflicts. In addition, they provide information about and make referrals to appropriate social service agencies within the county.

Follow-up Services

Aroostook Mental Health Services, Inc.
c/o Community General Hospital
Green Street
Fort Fairfield, Maine 04742

Paraprofessionals help to assess whether clients are best suited for living within their former homes or in "foster homes," where healthy adults provide a normalized setting. The paraprofessionals provide consultation services to the foster parents when appropriate.

Central Bergen Mental Health Center
289 Market Street
Saddlebrook, New Jersey 07652

Paraprofessionals supply support services to clients living with other clients in apartments in community settings. These services are provided on a 24-hour basis for newly discharged patients.

Central Plains Comprehensive Community Mental Health and Mental Retardation Center
2601 Dimmitt Road
P. O. Box 578
Plainview, Texas 79072

Within each of six rural satellite centers, a paraprofessional is responsible for both screening and follow-up services. Assisted by appropriate supervision and backup support from a professional, the paraprofessionals provide screening services for state hospitals, public schools, and the courts.

The Counseling Center
43 Illinois Avenue
Bangor, Maine 04401

The program employs four paraprofessionals who specialize in providing follow-up services to clients discharged from institutions for the mentally retarded.

Hahnemann Community Mental Health Center
314 North Broad Street
Philadelphia, Pennsylvania 19102

Paraprofessionals offer consultation and training to undertrained staff members working in community-based boarding homes. The assistance is focused primarily on medication issues, diagnosis of psychological problems, and therapeutic activities for the residents. The paraprofessionals supplement these indirect services with some direct services for the nursing home residents who can benefit from assistance in securing jobs.

A paraprofessional is in charge of linking the community mental health center with the state hospitals that discharge clients to the center's catchment district. The paraprofessional teaches hospital staff members about predischarge planning and about aftercare services provided within the catchment district.

Prairie View Mental Health Center
East First Street
P. O. Box 467
Newton, Kansas 67114

The paraprofessionals who provide follow-up services to former state hospital patients are employed by the "Community Services Division" of the mental health center. In this role, paraprofessionals provide services to a variety of types of clients and facilities. The services include socialization groups and activity groups that can be attended free of charge by former mental patients *and* by other residents of the catchment area.

West Central Community Services Center, Inc.
1125 6th Street, S.E.
Willmar, Minnesota 56201

The follow-up program provides mobile clinics to serve former state hospital patients in a large rural catchment area.

Inpatient Services

Connecticut Mental Health Center
P. O. Box 1842
34 Park Street
New Haven, Connecticut 06508

Paraprofessionals and other staff members make use of a "problem-oriented" record system for purposes of diagnosis and treatment planning.

Palo Verde Hospital
801 S. Prudence Road
Tucson, Arizona 85710

At Palo Verde, treatment teams of professional and paraprofessional personnel work with units composed of eight to twelve clients. Two rooms have been set aside at the hospital to house a closed circuit television system. The two cameras and video record/playback system are used for both treatment programs and training activities.

Tulsa Community Mental Health Center
1620 East 12th Street
Tulsa, Oklahoma 74120

Emphasis is placed on provision of a "normalized" environment involving planning by clients, an absence of staff uniforms, and considerable time spent out of doors. Diagnoses focus on functional skills rather than on degree of sickness.

Outpatient Services

Hahnemann Community Mental Health Center
314 North Broad Street
Philadelphia, Pennsylvania 19102

The outpatient services provided by this center are described in Appendix A: Supervision, in this volume.

North Central Community Mental Health Center
Beury Building—3701 North Broad Street
Philadelphia, Pennsylvania 19140

Paraprofessionals provide a variety of therapy and other intervention services for low-income minority clients in mental health centers and community locations.

North Richmond Mental Health Center
35 Austin Place
New York, New York 10307
     Appropriately trained paraprofessionals provide very long-term therapy services to individual clients.

Northern Arizona Comprehensive Guidance Center, Inc.
611 N. Leroux
Flagstaff, Arizona 86001
     A satellite clinic on the Apache Reservation provides short-term crisis-oriented services appropriate to the local American Indian culture. A majority of the staff members (including the director) are Indian paraprofessionals.

South Santa Clara County Community Mental Health Center
287 Leavesley Road
P. O. Box 1744
Gilroy, California 95020
     Spanish-speaking paraprofessionals provide therapy, outreach, and advocacy services to Chicano persons, including migrant farm workers.

Western Psychiatric Institute
3811 O'Hara Street
Pittsburgh, Pennsylvania 15261
     The institute operates specialty clinics in which clients receive outpatient services geared to particular types of mental health problems.

Screening Services

     The descriptions provided below portray three programs based in mental health centers and two programs based in autonomous public agencies. These latter programs implement strategies to reduce or prevent crime; they are included in this listing because some of the procedures used are potentially transferable to mental health centers.

PROGRAMS BASED IN MENTAL HEALTH CENTERS

Midtown Community Mental Health Clinic
960 Locke Street
Indianapolis, Indiana 46202
     Paraprofessionals provide screening services within the emergency room of a hospital for clients arrested for disorderly conduct. While only some of these clients are candidates for inpatient treatment, a number of the remaining clients are in need of other types of mental health services.

Upper Montgomery Community Mental Health Center
Montgomery General Hospital
18101 Prince Philip Drive
Olney, Maryland 20832
     Paraprofessionals are involved in providing consultation services to court-referred petitioners who have requested that the court consider the advisability of inpatient

treatment for a client. When appropriate, the paraprofessionals make recommendations to the petitioners for appropriate alternative routes for handling crisis situations.

Washtenaw County Community Mental Health Center
2929 Plymouth Road
Ann Arbor, Michigan 48105

Paraprofessionals provide home-based screening services for clients, and provide diagnostic examinations, treatment recommendations, and consultation services to a wide variety of social service agencies.

PROGRAMS BASED IN OTHER PUBLIC AGENCIES

Community-Based Corrections Program
Fifth Judicial District Department of Court Services
1000 College Avenue
Des Moines, Iowa 50314

A Law Enforcement Assistance Administration "exemplary" project, the Community-Based Corrections Program is designed to improve the quality of justice for defendants. Emphasizing social (e.g., jobs, education) rather than psychological factors, the program provides four alternatives for qualifying adult defendants. These alternatives are: release on own recognizance; pretrial supervised release; probation; and residence at a correctional facility offering work and educational release. Paraprofessionals help staff in all four programs. Defendants with more severe mental health problems are referred to various treatment agencies, including the area community mental health center and the area state mental hospital. For a manual describing the program in detail, write:

U.S. Department of Justice
Law Enforcement Assistance Administration
Washington, D.C. 20531

Volunteer Probation Counselor Program
129 North Tenth Street
Lincoln, Nebraska 68508

A Law Enforcement Assistance Administration "exemplary" project, the Volunteer Counselor Program employs paraprofessional probation officers to provide direct services to young offenders (ages 15–25) and to train and supervise community volunteers to provide additional services. The probation counselors provide counseling services, handle crises, and teach educational classes for special populations (e.g., petty larceny offenders, drunken drivers). The volunteer counselors are carefully screened, trained, and then matched with youthful offenders. They can provide counseling and crisis intervention services for up to a year. In an experimental study, the recidivism rate among program enrollees during a one-year period was 15%; the rate for a comparable group of control subjects was 64%. For a manual describing this program in detail, write:

U.S. Department of Justice
Law Enforcement Assistance Administration
Washington, D.C. 20531

INDEX